The
WELLNESS LIFESTYLE

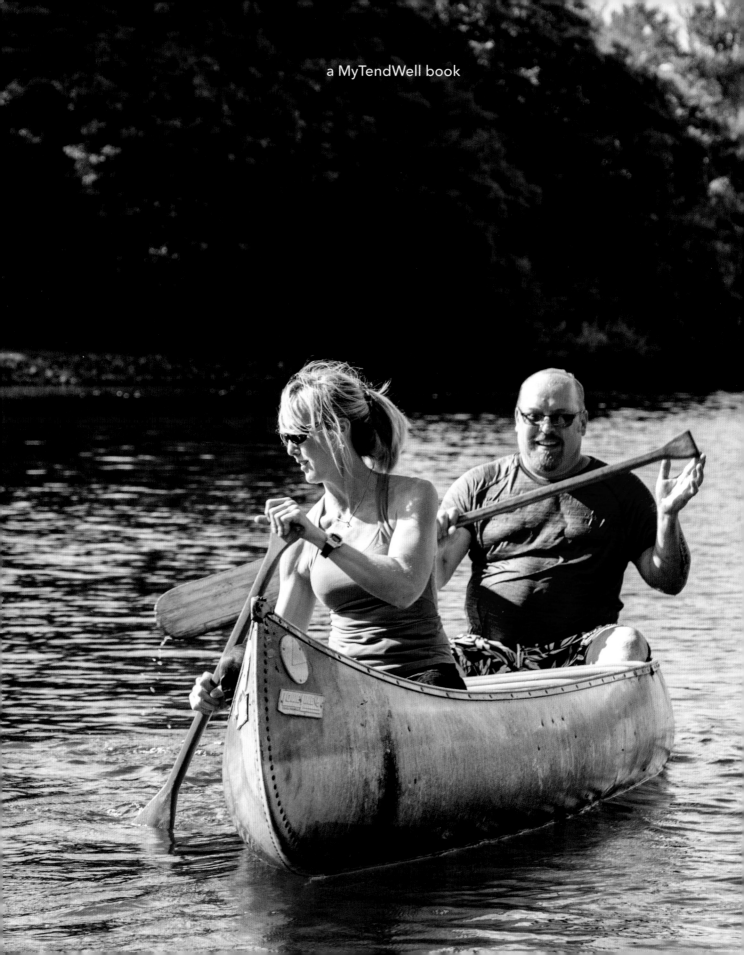

a MyTendWell book

The WELLNESS LIFESTYLE

A Chef's Recipe for Real Life

DANIEL ORR *&*
KELLY JO BAUTE, PhD

RED ⚡ LIGHTNING BOOKS

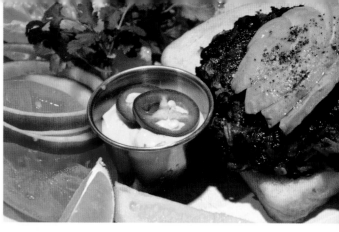

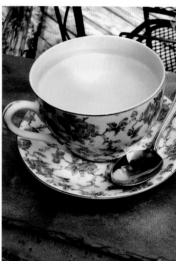

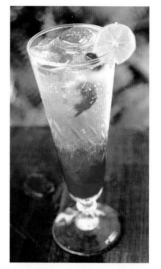

This book is a publication of

Red Lightning Books
1320 East 10th Street
Bloomington, Indiana 47405 USA

redlightningbooks.com

Manufactured in China

Cataloging information is available
from the Library of Congress.

ISBN 978-1-68435-059-9 (paperback)
ISBN 978-1-68435-056-8 (ebook)

1 2 3 4 5   23 22 21 20 19 18

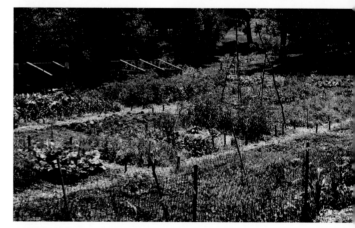

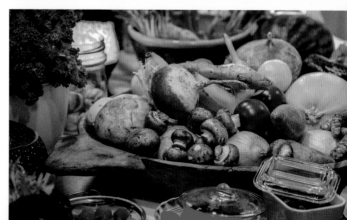

CONTENTS

The Wellness Lifestyle: A Chef's Recipe for Real Life is a marriage of food and fitness and was written to assist those obsessed with food and struggling with daily physical activity. *Who qualifies?* Anyone who collects cookbooks, buys quick-fix exercise books, watches cooking shows and weight-loss programs, or makes it a priority in life to dine in the newest, trendiest restaurants, all while struggling with the buttons, zippers, and snaps in the morning when getting dressed for work on Monday. Chefs, who are obviously obsessed with food, will also love this book. The guests in our restaurants eat our cooking occasionally; we are tempted by bacon fat, *foie gras*, and caviar every day. Chefs eat, drink, and sleep their cuisine 24/7 and must learn how to balance their pleasures and their pounds. People who love to eat, professional chefs, and amateur cooks will find the book educational, entertaining, and inspirational. People who need to learn how to move their bodies will find Chef D and Dr. K's plan appealing and easy to fit into everyday life. *The Wellness Lifestyle: A Chef's Recipe for Real Life* is a recording of a successful shift in lifestyle by one of America's best chefs. It's a fulfilling "recipe" for people interested in losing weight without losing out on one of life's greatest pleasures: food! Chef D wants to teach you how to "sauté off the pounds" (SOTP) with this new style of healthy cooking he has developed for the MyTendWell program.

"Break the routine and get on the regime!"
—*Real Food* by Daniel Orr

The Wellness Lifestyle: A Chef's Recipe for Real Life was born in the Caribbean through a series of twenty articles written for *The Anguillian*, the national newspaper of Anguilla, the island where Chef Orr cooked in 2004 and 2005. In his column, "Eating My Words," Chef D shared his adventures in dieting and healthy eating in the kitchens of CuisinArt Resort and Spa with the people of Anguilla. These articles make up the basis for the lifestyle plan. Chef D invited Dr. Kelly Jo Baute to bring the book full circle by developing the wellness programming of the exercise material to ensure it is the most up-to-date information and that the nutrition plan is a safe way of eating.

The numbers of chronic, and costly, health issues are skyrocketing. Type 2 diabetes is on the rise, and by the year 2025, two-thirds of the US population will be diagnosed with a debilitating disease—a completely preventable disease. Dr. K stands behind this lifestyle philosophy for preventing disease and improving overall quality of life. Families that adopt this active, healthy, and positive lifestyle will be giving their children a wellness upbringing.

This has been a long and winding road for Chef D, and he continues to work on his goal of having a healthier lifestyle and control over all the temptations that life throws at him. There have been many detours and roadblocks along the way: opening a new business, the roller-coaster economy, family issues, life, death, personal challenges, outside pressures. You know—life. Staying on track is one of the biggest issues with making long-term lifestyle changes. Chef D and Dr. K understand this and have created a lifestyle plan that moves you toward your goal, even if it takes longer than you would hope. It's like riding a bike, right? If you fall off, it is easier to get back on if you know what you are doing, even if you have a few Band-Aids on your wounds. Those battle scars make us who we are. Come join us on the ride!

The *Wellness Lifestyle* and the "Sautéing Off the Pounds" Kitchen are, in the proverbial nutshell:

- Balancing protein, complex carbohydrates, and healthy fats.

- Eating more local, organic, and naturally produced foods

- Consuming more complex carbohydrates and fewer refined carbohydrates, such as white bread, muffins, crackers, and bagels

- Consuming more fruits, vegetables, fiber, legumes, and whole grains

- Reducing consumption of sweets, sugars, carbonated beverages, juices, and caffeine

- Consuming more fish high in omega-3 fatty acids, leaner grass-fed and pastured meats, and eliminating processed meat and meat produced with hormones

- Eliminating processed foods with additives, GMOs, and coloring agents

- Reducing/eliminating snack foods, frozen foods, and canned foods

- Reducing intake of saturated fats while increasing intake of unsaturated fats

- Eliminating consumption of trans and hydrogenated fats totally

- Decreasing portion sizes of proteins and increasing whole grains, fresh vegetables, and fruits

- Reducing heavy alcohol intake

- Drinking the proper amount of water per day depending on body size and amount of movement

- Increasing healthy and safe movement, and setting a date with yourself for some type of moving daily

- Most important, sharing physical activity, food, wine, and the pleasures of the table with the ones you love

ACKNOWLEDGMENTS

Chef D and Dr. K would like to thank families and friends for their support and encouragement during the development of the MyTendWell Lifestyle Plan and the writing of this book.

Big thanks to Ali Sohrabi, the GM at FARMbloomington Restaurant, and his hard working FOH managers. Chef Chris Hoppie and sous chefs Ryan Johnson, Chelsi Field, and J. Brandon Shepard—you all are the best. Thanks/gracias to all the FARMhands for their support and care. "Teamwork makes the dream work." They all stepped up and allowed Chef D to take the time to finish this tome.

Many meetings and work sessions were at FARMbloomington Restaurant, and the FARMhands went above and beyond the call of duty. Great food and service! Chef D's "work wife" Ginny Henderson was, and is, always amazing—even with her poor taste in music . . .

As always, Mary Lu Orr (a.k.a. Mom) has put up with our shenanigans. She has allowed us to take over her kitchen, home, and gardens for months on end. She has tasted the food, corrected our English, done the dishes, made quick trips to the market, and looked over the fact that there is a giant monitor and snaking computer cords taking over her breakfast nook.

Thanks to the local farmers who work so hard to put the wonderful products in our larder; we would not be able to eat as well without you.

We would also like to thank David Porter for his enthusiasm for life, countless technological tips and guidance, and photography and videography contributions. A thank you also goes out to Ellen Olmstead for her exceptional contributions of friendship, photography, and videography.

Additional thanks go to Liz Porter, Mary Beth Porter, Peter Magurean III, John B. Shea, PhD, Cindy Bradley, Linda Oblack, Krista Hill, and others.

And finally to Ashley Runyon, David Hulsey, Peggy Solic, and everyone at Red Lightning Press for taking our beautiful baby, sending it through grammar school, and giving it a facelift—it wouldn't be as pretty with all the wrinkles.

Chef D:

Many thanks to Elizabeth DiMeo who helped me get started on this project many years ago while I was still in Manhattan; her passion and knowledge were inspiring and instrumental. Now many years and a roller-coaster ride up and down the bathroom scales later, I'm happy to have found some answers. Things have changed on the landscape of health and wellness. Thanks for getting me on the path.

A big "meow out" to the two kitties in my life, the Tuxedo Twins, Cooper and Conner.

Thank you, Christopher Brown.

Dr. K:

Dr. K would like to, first and foremost, thank her two boys, Levi and Kyle. They are the ones who always give the most when their mom is working on her projects. All I do is for them.

Dr. K would also like to thank her mom, Shelley, as all she does is for *her* children. And, finally, to Dr. John Shea for his exceptional academic training and *poor* professional advice.

The
WELLNESS
LIFESTYLE

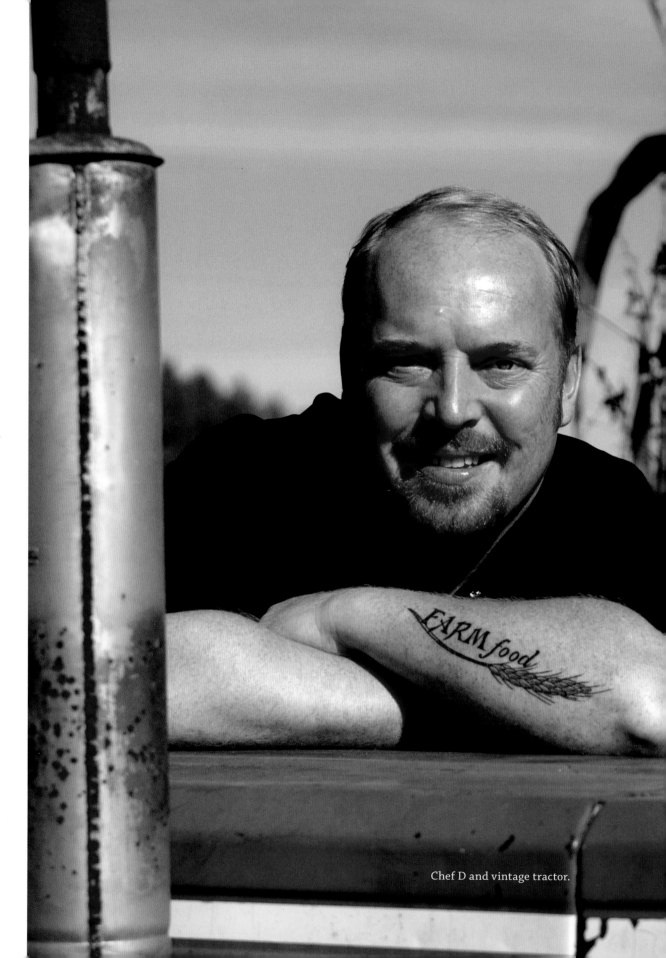
Chef D and vintage tractor.

1 The MyTendWell Lifestyle Plan

CHEF D'S JOURNEY

Today is the first day of the rest of your life. Eat it up!

The classic image of a chef is a round, jolly man with one hand's finger in the pot and the other hand holding a wine glass. That guy usually dies around the age of 45 owing $500K to the bank! But that is the way chefs have been for hundreds of years until those food nazis and health authorities came up with the "fake news" that eating properly gives you a longer and more productive life. The problem is that the facts have been scientifically demonstrated and now most of us can no longer have our "alternative facts." A healthy eating and movement regime has truly become food for thought for us all. Death and taxes I can deal with. The two words any bon vivant shudders over are *diet* and *exercise*!

In the past, restaurants built a wall, a huge and beautiful wall, between the dining room and the kitchen, which was a great way to keep those crazy chefs from immigrating into the dining room. Homes were also built with a separate room for the kitchen where the "woman's work" was done, disallowing others to see (or hear) the throwing of pots and pans, the dropping of the turkey on the floor, or the quick recovery of said turkey within the "30-second rule." In restaurants, waiters and busboys bowed and looked the other way. Now the home kitchen has become the heart of the home, the true living room

of the house. And the chef, who often works in an open kitchen, has become a media darling who must keep temper and waistline in check. There was once a saying that you should never trust a skinny chef because he must not taste his own cooking. Nowadays a chef needs to have a personal trainer as well as a spiritual adviser to keep in shape both physically and mentally. The competition for restaurant space, TV airtime, brand naming, and publishing is so intense that the poor artist in the kitchen, stirring his or her sauces and cooking clients' food, is all too often forgotten. Becoming a celebrity chef, much like a sports star or supermodel, is now something kids aspire to achieve. When I was a kid, the chef was the help.

The celebrity chef phenomenon began in France in the late 1970s and early 1980s with talents such as Paul Bocuse, Roger Vergé, and Michel Guérard. Americans were drawn to France after devouring Julia Child's and James Beard's cookbooks and TV appearances. As meat-and-potato Americans traveled throughout Europe, they discovered a new appreciation for cooking and eating. The French/European passion for food and drink taught Yankees eating to live is not as fun as living to eat. This lifestyle stressed quality over quantity and included seasonal appreciation for the best ingredients available. But, being Americans, we took this to the extreme, consuming vast amounts of calories during our 24/7 way of life, and now 40 percent of us are obese.

Inspired by my personal and constant battles of the bulge, I have always looked for healthy things to eat, both on duty at the restaurant and at home entertaining myself and/or friends. I've taken notes on these dishes because friends always ask for recipes, especially if the dish is easy and healthful. One of my own rules for healthy eating is that it has gotta be good. I don't want to miss the fat I love so dearly—so healthy food has gotta be kick-ass. I know good food, and I am not one to punish myself by staring into a bowl of plain steamed cabbage. But if you jazz that bowl up with the inspiration of a chef, that cabbage can be glorious. Add some citrus, a drop of sesame oil, Chinese chili paste, and some diced tofu and you've got something better than any white box delivery! Plus you have the added bonus of knowing what is *really* in it. And let's not make FAT the criminal; fat is an important part of any meal. It just has to be the right kind of fat and in the correct proportion. Essential fats allow for the proper absorption of fat-soluble vitamins into the body, provide the building blocks for cell structures and hormones, and are instrumental in other bodily tasks such as immune and visual functioning. So, let's stop bullying our friend: FAT, we love you!

I had been preaching healthy eating, but the time came to eat my own words. After working on the Guastavino project in Manhattan for four years and being in Manhattan when the twin towers fell, I slipped into a funk: I stopped working out, I split with the love of my life (I thought at the time . . .), and I gained 40 lb. I knew it was time for a change, and I knew I had the skill and knowledge to make it happen. The problem was the lack of *self-love* and *motivation*. Sadness and loneliness had me feeling as if I were drifting away from my dream and my focus; but, as things will do, a new door opened for me.

It was then that I moved to the beautiful Caribbean island of Anguilla, British West Indies, for a change of pace and stress level. I decided to get things under control and to have a good time doing it. That was years ago, and the result is this book, designed to help others who love food eat smartly and with gusto and flavor. By introducing a new vocabulary of ingredients, easy techniques, and satisfying comforts for people who have eaten "too well" and now want to eat better, it is my hope that foodies who read this book will become more interested in what food does in the body and not just what it does on the palate. Chefs have spread the word on food quality and artistry; now the next logical step is the consideration of nutrition and the offering of healthy alternatives to their guests. At CuisinArt Resort and Spa in Anguilla I had the opportunity to offer these findings at our Spa Grill, 24/7 RAW juice bar, as well as in the Santorini fine Caribbean and Greek inspired dining. I have always offered healthy foods in the restaurants I've run, but this was a chance to take it to the next level. *Regime cuisine* is what I called it in my first book, *Real Food*. Simply put, it is lighter dishes for a healthier lifestyle. I had even based a wildly popular seven-course degustation menu (a fancy French name for a chef's tasting menu) at the fine-dining room at The Resort using the hydroponically and organically grown produce from the property in nutritionally balanced recipes. That setting is truly a chef's paradise. Now, back home again in Indiana, I have continued this at my own restaurant, FARMbloomington.

Everyone faces temptations, but imagine a restaurateur who loves food and is surrounded by it 24/7. Picture the poor chef at the market all morning and at the stove all afternoon and night. How can he not succumb to luscious bites? It is nigh impossible to adore something and to hold it close without having a taste of it. One of my favorite things is my Parmesan-dusted French fries with citrus zest, chili flakes, and turmeric aioli. I was tasting them way too often and the pounds just started adding up. The home cook is also bombarded and haunted by food, from junk food on the airwaves to more nutritional offerings. One must learn to balance desire and indulgence. It was for this reason I decided to create this regime of healthy eating. Although I usually get concerned about my weight because of vanity, it is certainly more important to eat smartly for less visual, more vital reasons.

So, the eating part is a challenge in itself; fitting in a workout—WTF . . . I couldn't make the time. Opening a new restaurant, and struggling back from a ski injury, was overwhelming. And to top that off, I was dragging around IV antibiotics to fight the MRSA infection I contracted during surgery to repair my ACL. Exercise was just not possible, and, by the time it was, I was out of habit and failed to get it into my daily routine. Starting FARM restaurant was a lot of work, and it still is, but its success was my priority—my health wasn't. By the time I realized I had gained all of this weight, I could not get motivated to lose it. Dr. K helped with building a schedule, a routine that *I* could handle, that I could fit into *my* day.

DR. K'S JOURNEY

Just as Chef D struggled keeping weight off, I've had struggles with keeping weight, or rather muscle, on. Just over five years ago, I was diagnosed with breast cancer. My first mammogram! It was a devastating journey. I experienced numerous difficulties along the way. A botched reconstruction, nearly every side effect chemotherapy has to offer, one surgery or procedure after another—10 in under 5 years. Wellness? What wellness? It seemed gone and sometimes lost forever. I could no longer move my body as I once could and knew how to move it. Movement had been my foundation. Movement was my stress reliever, my recreation, my study, and my way of life and living. Instead, I hurt. I couldn't lift my arms or move my neck and shoulders. And when I repeatedly asked when it would get better, my doctor said, "Look, in my world, at the end of the

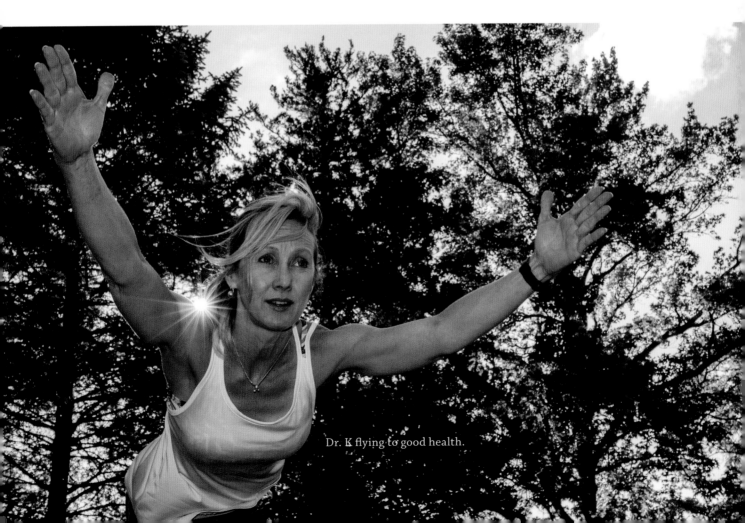

Dr. K flying to good health.

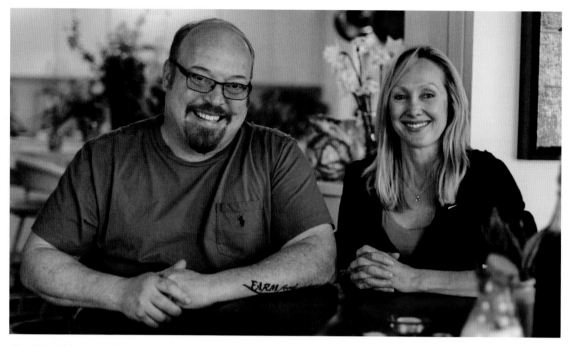

Chef D and Dr. K welcome you to MyTendWell.

day, I am a plastic surgeon and I'm concerned with looks, not pain, and we have good visual results." That is verbatim. It was like a dagger. And his solution—pain management! "Yes, let's send you to yet another doctor to give you medications and nerve blocks." Well, I've witnessed that approach from the sidelines, watching clients being taken down one path after another—rarely if ever finding relief.

Fortunately, there are good doctors out there—straight shooters only another would love. "You need different implants. Those don't fit your body. They look awful," says a kind face through half-grinning teeth—not a grin of joy but disappointment at the whole situation, as if she were asking herself, "Why could she not have been told this earlier?" And this doctor knew what she was talking about. She gave me two names; I called the first, and onward to better physical and emotional wellness was I. So needed was a revision that the moment I woke in the recovery room, the first words out of my mouth, as I placed my hands on my chest, were, "I can already feel the difference." The relief was

immediate! Gone was that discomfort, that pain I could not shed with physical therapy or with muscle relaxers. It was wonderful. I began moving again—moving and getting my body back, rebuilding my wellness, moving along the continuum toward optimal functioning, and trying to get back the muscle—and the strength—that was GONE.

It was at this time Chef D and Dr. K met and began working together and developing the concept of MyTendWell. Ironically, as Chef D was trying to learn how best to understand his eating patterns and exercise behaviors, essentially dealing with food, Dr. K was trying to move again, while building a company that teaches movement and wellness. Both were dealing with their own passions, food and movement. Chef D had begun constructing the majority of these recipes in Anguilla. He saw Dr. K's work, her knowledge of movement, health, and wellness, as a basis for a perfect collaboration. And collaborate they have. The MyTendWell Lifestyle Plan is a comprehensive wellness program that teaches you along the way, allowing you to make a lifestyle change, not a quick fix. Wellness is holistic. Wellness is the integration and balance of multiple dimensions. The MyTendWell Lifestyle Plan is focused on the following eight dimensions: social, occupational, intellectual, physical, emotional, spiritual, environmental, and nutritional.

Wellness doesn't have a finish line—it is a continuum. It is a lifelong pursuit in which you work toward higher levels of wellness or optimal functioning. Importantly, it is *work* that moves you into higher levels of functioning. Thus, in order to achieve optimal levels of functioning, follow the plan's Five Steps to Wellness.

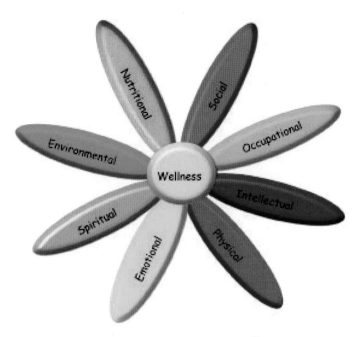

The MyTendWell wellness flower.

THE MyTendWell LIFESTYLE PLAN: FIVE STEPS TO WELLNESS

Step 1: Identify where you are within Prochaska and DiClemente's Model of Stages of Change (chapter 2).

Step 2: Write out your SMART Goals (chapter 3).

Step 3: Start recording daily entries for 30 days (minimum) in your log (chapter 3).

Step 4: Assemble your Toolbox and your Pantry (chapter 3).

Step 5: Schedule your physical activity like an appointment and plan your meals for the week ahead.

Now do it!

mytendwell.com

By following the MyTendWell Lifestyle Plan, you are taking ownership of your wellness plan. You have thought and worked through your plan in order to be successful in achieving optimal wellness. Chef D and Dr. K have learned how to fill their MyTendWell flowers to build total wellness. They have battled through their health challenges and have come through just fine. They have also developed from a combination of expertise in their respective fields a lifestyle program that is fun and rewarding. MyTendWell Lifestyle Plan is easy to follow and sets you up for success. You will be tending to your wellness, tending to your life.

An interesting paradox revealed itself between their individual wellness plans. Just as Chef D has struggled with fitting in exercise (and balanced meals), Dr. K was really struggling to fit in good meals. Having clients early in the morning and classes or clients at lunch and in the evenings was really disrupting her diet. Dr. K was not eating enough, eating on the fly, and typically eating quick foods, such as smoothies, fruit, and sandwiches/wraps. But not enough. Dr. K had lost a lot of weight during

DIET AND EXERCISE

The word **diet** actually refers to what an organism is consuming on a regular basis. We misuse the word *diet* by using it to refer to a restriction in what we (can) consume.

The word **exercise** is often misused as well. *Exercise* refers to planned physical movement structured to address a specific physical function or need such as improving cardiovascular function.

Chef D and Dr. K want you to rethink these words and their meanings and consider not thinking about restricting what you are eating but rather expanding what you are eating. And consider thinking not about an hour-long bout of exercise but rather about random or intermittent physical activity throughout the day. Whereas exercise is used to describe planned and structured bouts of physical movement, *physical activity* refers to all physical movement, from cleaning the house to hiking a trail. Dr. K says our biology/physiology adapted to a lifestyle of intermittent bouts of physical activity and that long periods of sitting and not moving affect more than caloric expenditure. Read more on the benefits of intermittent physical activity in later sections.

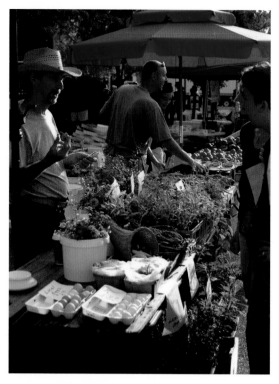

Supporting the Bloomington Farmers' Market as well as getting nutritional, social, and environmental wellness.

cancer treatments/therapies, and as she was getting busier and more active with her wellness and ergonomics company, she was not getting enough nutrition and lost even more muscle. So, she put the MyTendWell Lifestyle Plan into action. And guess what? It worked—she added muscle, which left her stronger and feeling much more energetic. Her job, as do all other jobs, requires energy, with some left over. Getting and staying fit helps provide that abundance of energy to get you through your day and still have some energy to spare. See, it's like she had been telling her clients for years, "It takes energy to make energy." In other words, you've got to put a little in to get a little out—kinda primin' the pump, so to speak.

Adopting a total wellness approach for a healthy lifestyle includes building an environment that supports and sustains this philosophy. When Dr. K began working with Chef D, they first discussed the environments in which he lives, works, and plays. Investigations into physical activity behaviors have demonstrated that the environment has an effect on physical activity and dietary factors. Her experiences working with individuals in wellness programming for the past 20-plus years indicated that home and work settings either encourage or discourage movement. If you work in an environment that promotes sitting, you will sit. Conversely, standing workstations promote standing. However, neither of those behaviors is movement. Movement *is* the substrate of physical activity (Malina 2008), and persistent physical activity *is* the behavior that promotes health. So just as Dr. K was having a hard time fitting in *good* meals, Chef D was having a hard time fitting in movement. The MyTendWell Lifestyle Plan worked for him as well. He adjusted his work schedule so he had consistent days off, and we created a workout that fit his schedule. And guess what? It worked.

Dr. K has worked within the wellness industry for nearly 25 years. She has seen the trends in exercise classes, weight loss programs, drinks, and supplements. The bottom line is this: quick fixes and programs of restricting foods or training at high intensities are not sustainable. Just as the world is searching for sustainable practices in agricultural, energy production, and building

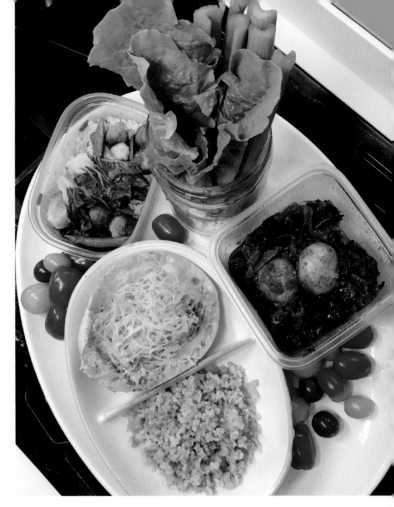

Prepping your nutritional wellness with Chef D's Meal Plan.

COOK YOUR OWN MEALS

People are now eating more meals out than in for the first time in history. But what are they eating? Typically it's fast food that is produced for quantity (in a short time) as opposed to quality. The compromise for quantity over quality is problematic. We need to have more healthful choices as well as to learn new ways to prepare foods that are high quality and will have a positive impact on health. Motivate yourself to cook more meals. Rethink your life and manage your days in order to make the time to nourish your body with healthy foods and tasty meals. Chef D has created sample meal plans to help get you started.

structures, you, too, are searching for a health program that is sustainable for you and your life. This is the crux of the MyTendWell Lifestyle Plan. Chef D and Dr. K know the importance of reflecting on your life and developing a mindfulness about it. That is an ability to step back and reflect, view with an open mind, and figure out what went wrong and what could be more successful. We are all going to have ups and downs. We have the ability to survive the ride and level ourselves off and to get our bearings so we can get back on track. Dr. K had a lot of track to cover to get back to a healthy body. Chemotherapy is a nice name for poison. That's right, poison. Just the right concoction of chemicals to kill stuff off—good and bad. Some chemotherapy drugs kill off all respiring cells. Some chemotherapy drugs kill specific cells—these are targeted chemotherapy drugs. These are wonderful in that they do not kill off other cells, like hair cells, and thus, targeted therapy is a little kinder to your body. Dr. K had two old-fashioned chemotherapy drugs and one targeted chemotherapy drug. And just like other chemicals, chemo drugs stay in your body for a while. Thus, you deal with the effects for a time after you've stopped taking them. Take care of people you may know in chemotherapy and radiation treatment; they need some TLC. She did get stronger and her energy back—it took time and persistence. Until then, the lack of energy was like lumbering around in another's cumbersome body. But, "it takes energy to make energy." So she put in the energy and got back *her* body. And so did Chef D. They have the pep back in their step. *Persistent application toward one steadfast goal.*

DIET?
A DIRTY FOUR-LETTERED WORD

Diet, that dirty four-letter word, plays a primary role in determining one's level of health and wellness. Remember: diet is not what you don't eat, it is really what you do eat. Diet should be used as a noun not a verb. Let's replace the word

diet with the phrases *healthy eating* or *healthy regime*. Proper dietary practices can prevent a wide range of diseases by helping to maintain ideal body weight. This emphasis on what we eat and how we move will help us in achieving and maintaining good health. This will come with a wide range of changes in the way most people approach food and that other hated word, *exercise*.

Over the past several decades, chefs have influenced our diets by reopening the door to cooking with fresh herbs, using seasonal food, and introducing international flavors. This has been done in the realm of great restaurants and TV cooking shows that tantalize and inspire even the most timid eaters. Trends, such as the slow-food movement in Europe (now worldwide), which emphasizes a back-to-basics approach to the growing and eating of traditional foods, and sustainable cuisine, which advocates reduced exposure to pesticides and herbicides through organic farming and near-to-farm source marketing, help change the ways we think about food. And local agriculture is supported by these programs. Even the weekly trip to the farmers' market is not only reviving our taste buds and supporting community farmers but is also helping to reduce the habit of relying

WHAT IS OVERWEIGHT? WHAT IS OBESE?

Body mass index (BMI) is typically used to classify weight and health status. BMI is your body weight (in kilograms) divided by your height (in meters, squared)

Example:
150 lb. = 68.04 kg / 5 ft., 7 in. (67 in.) = 1.702 sq. m = 2.897m² = BMI = 23.5 kg/m²

Body mass index (BMI) ranges:
<18.5 = underweight
18.5 to <25 = normal
25 to <30 = overweight
30 and higher = obese

CURRENT US STATISTICS FOR OBESITY

Adult Obesity (BMI = ≥30, male and female)
age 20-39 = 36.3%
age 40-59 = 40.2%
age 60 and over = 37.0%

Child/Adolescent Obesity
age 2-5 = 8.9%
age 6-11 = 17.5%
age 12-19 = 20.5%

Data sources: National Health and Nutrition Examination Survey 1999-2014. CDC National Center for Health Statistics Data Brief, No. 219, November 2015.

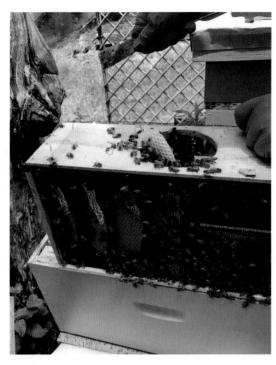

Caring for the environment by caring for bees.

misleading to many consumers: low-fat foods that appear to be good for you can be high in calories, while many so-called health foods are overprocessed and less healthful than advertisers might admit. Foods often don't taste real or good, and you can forget about *really good*. I have always believed you should eat the real thing: eat the butter, eat the cream, eat the chocolate, but eat it as a small celebration and enjoy it to the fullest. Chew it, let it melt in your mouth, enjoy the experience, but do it with control, by monitoring your portions, balancing your calories with getting the right amount of nutrients and being active—daily!

Another big concern is coming from industrial farming. Our animals are mostly fed an unnatural diet meant to have them grow quickly and to enormous sizes. They are kept in confined areas not allowing them a life of pastures and sunshine. The cage- or feedlot-raised animals

on unhealthy mass-produced foods. It is a lot of fun to get out there and rub elbows with humanity and to get an old family recipe or two from some of the farmer-sellers.

Despite the positive developments in our approach to food and nutrition, obesity is in epidemic proportions both in the United States and throughout the Western world, especially among our children. Children haven't much say or choice in their nutrition. We parents/guardians are to blame for their nutrition, activity level, and subsequent health status—overweight and experiencing what have been typically midlife adult-onset diseases (cardiovascular disease, diabetes). Increased portion sizes at home, in school cafeterias, and in restaurants; processed convenience foods from grocery stores; and the reliance on fast-food chain eateries contribute to this trend of overeating. Food manufacturers continue to produce foods with additives, coloring agents, and preservatives that can contribute to food allergies and a host of other health problems. The corporate marketing of food is

GENETICALLY MODIFIED ORGANISMS

Genetically modified organisms (**GMOs**) are genetically engineered, or modified, in labs to enhance the productivity of a plant or animal and make it less susceptible to diseases and even tolerant of certain substances or chemicals, such as weed killers. For example, Roundup-ready soybeans, corn, or wheat are genetically engineered to withstand applications of Roundup, or glyphosate.

There is concern that genetically engineered or modified organisms are harmful to our health, although there is no evidence suggesting so. However, critics argue that the use of GMOs is so recent, less than 20 years, that it is not nearly enough time to see whether they affect us.

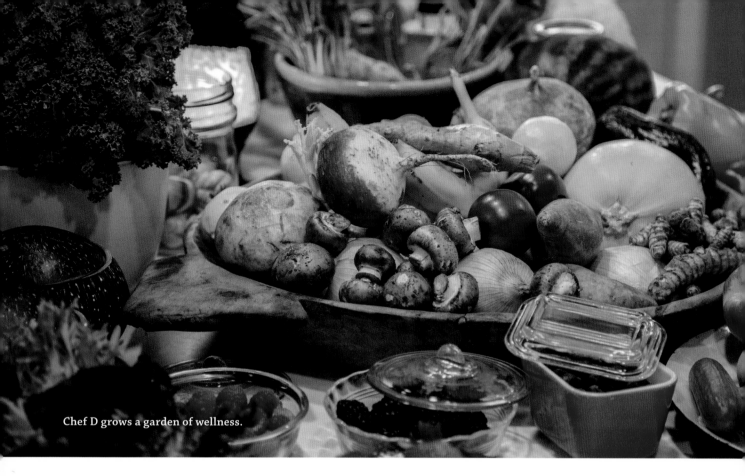

Chef D grows a garden of wellness.

MyTendWell CHALLENGE

Feed the Birds . . . Flower Toppings

Your pretty flowers fed you with joy and happiness as they bloomed and drew butterflies to your garden. Repurpose those beautiful flowers from spring, summer, and fall to feed the birds. Coneflower (*Echinacea purpurea*) is a hearty and lovely perennial flower and is also great at fighting bacterial and viral infections.

So don't be so quick to cut those dead flowers down and toss them in the street for city pickup. Let them stand and watch the American goldfinches flock to your yard. When the seed heads are gone, toss the stalks, stems, and foliage into your compost pile.

are so closely packed that they must be fed a constant diet of antibiotics and chemicals just to keep them alive long enough to reach the slaughterhouse. And then they are processed in large factories that often are not kept up to the sanitary standards we demand.

Our fruits and vegetables are grown variety by variety on large farms designed more for the planting and harvesting machines than for the quality of produce. This creates large areas of monoculture where only one crop is grown for miles and miles. The lack of variety and the short time of a solo crop's (monoculture) pollination window have caused havoc among honeybees and other animals and insects that depend on a whole season of food supply for them to thrive. Top that off with pesticides and herbicides, GMOs, loss of varieties of produce, nutritional loss caused by long-term storage and shipping, and we are left with a sad situation on our plates both in restaurants and on our home tables.

BENEFITS OF GARDENING

Try growing at least some of your food. You will know what you are eating and you will be addressing your environmental wellness. Further, research is showing that gardens and gardening provide therapeutic effects. Consider the time you spend gardening as a retreat or a break that allows you to downshift and go to your garden space, a space that is typically tranquil and provides a distraction from other tasks. Distraction hypothesis has been investigated in studies of physical activity and mental health, and findings suggest that a distraction from other thoughts, tasks, and so on, is beneficial and may serve as a time-out from stressful situations. Gardening is a task that allows you to focus intently and forget about the other stuff that might be weighing on you. You can leave the phone inside, listen to the sounds of the garden, and enjoy the little things you are growing. It's a positive activity that provides positive outcomes—fresh produce and relaxation—accompanied by nature's lovely birdsong and breezes.

Numerous dietary lifestyles such as the Atkins diet, the Zone diet, eating right for your blood type, the food pyramid, and even vegetarianism and veganism confuse people with their extremism and radical differences. The end result is that Americans still consume the Western diet—high in carbohydrates and saturated fat, and low in plant foods and fiber—that is contributing to this epidemic of obesity and ill health. We, as chefs, have the platform to help update the Western diet. (Think of the impact Julia Child had, bringing the art of French cooking to the United States, and she was a food writer and cook.) Chefs have the tools and the platform . . . and it isn't brain surgery. In fact we've already learned the way, with the incorporation of the Mediterranean diet into our menu planning. We need to plunge into the new century with all the knowledge and position we now have available to us.

The global appreciation of food is helping to contribute beneficial changes in our society, but it is the ambassadors for food—chefs, nutritionists, farmers, and supporters of good food—who must help define, drive, and educate the general population. Our goal is to make this adventurous and sometimes challenging new experience both fun and tasty. Dieting is a drag, but developing a healthy lifestyle is fun and rewarding. Yes, it will be a pain in the ass at times and you will fall off the organic wagon occasionally, but eating outrageously good food that takes less time to prepare than haute cuisine is a win/win.

Simple cooking and eating is the first step in beginning a program of good dietary practice and better health; as mentioned earlier, this is regime cuisine. And getting moving is right behind as a close second—this is the elixir for the body. These are two things you must do for yourself, every day, but think of them as your personal little treat or gift to yourself, not as disappointing chores that control you. You will love the food and movement recipes and what they do for your complete well-being. Learn the basics, then come up with your own versions, and, we hope, you will convert your family and friends. For the chefs out there, let's convert our customers along with ourselves. Make healthy food so good that guests won't know that they are reducing their caloric intake.

CHEF D: EXORCISING EXERCISE

I was a real gym bunny back in NYC in the late 1980s and the 1990s. Hell, I sometimes went to the gym twice a day and Rollerbladed to the

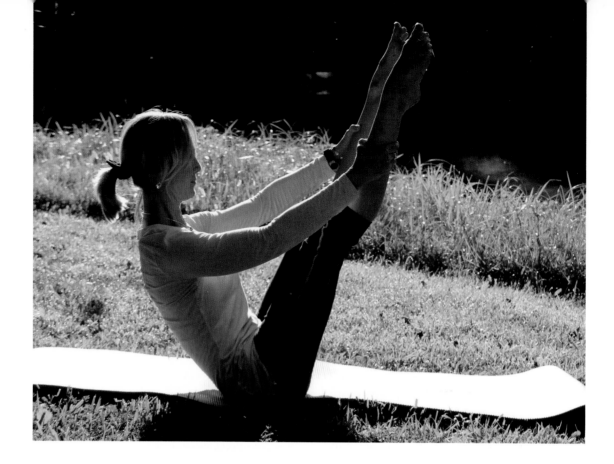

Union Square Farmers' Market, then up to 52nd Street for a 10-hour day at La Grenouille restaurant. But now, at 50-plus I'm finding it hard to get excited about exercise. The word brings me feelings of torture and pain. I have gone from an addiction to physical activity to a fear of it.

Of course, 15 years is a long time, but it has been more than age that has brought this on. One of the major reasons my weight went up was due to a knee surgery gone wrong. After I tore my ACL snow skiing, I had it repaired by a wonderful surgeon, but I got a staph infection in the wound and ended up having a walking IV for a month. Once the enormous swelling finally went down, I was left with a knee that couldn't do much. Through rehab and slow movement progressions, I am finally able to have a normal life most days but still have issues kneeling and with some movements. One thing for sure, no more Rollerblading.

Owning a business, especially in the food service industry, is tough on your personal schedule. The hours are always changing. Once-in-a-lifetime wedding events as well as last-minute catered parties pull you in every direction. Sous chefs give notice and someone has to cover the shift. A good client orders a dozen quiches for the next morning and no one else

> "You aren't going to get the butt you want by sitting on the one you have." —Unknown

has time to make them but you . . . and every penny counts in a nickel-and-dime business. The problem is that once you get off your routine, it is hard to get back on it. Just think how many exercise bikes have been turned into clothes trees.

What Dr. K has taught me is that movement is necessary. If you can't walk, it is hard to get anywhere. As we age we need to think less about exercise and more about healthy movement. In fact, exorcise the word *exercise* and get moving. Figure out enjoyable ways to fit movement into your daily life. It is less about trying to get a six-pack and more about not having a heart attack! At 50-plus and over 250 pounds it is hard to get back into the swing of pre- or postwork activities. When you don't like what you see in the mirror, it brings down your morale—I often turned to other activities that dulled the negative feelings I was having. Having wine or a cocktail and cooking something delicious for myself was much easier than hitting the gym.

The MyTendWell Lifestyle Plan breaks up the movement I need in my life into segments that I can fit in, just as anyone else can. Daily 15-minutes of muscle movement and 30- to 60-minutes of cardio movement, which I can add up over the course of the day, really is something you can do too. Dr. K's Back-in-Five station break movements can be fit into your 9–5 day and is much healthier than a coffee and doughnut break, not to mention a smoke break. If you can get a coworker to get on the program with you, it will make it more fun and that company will help you stay true to your new regime. Get friends and family involved and surround yourself with "Yes, you can!" people. There will be people who are close to you who don't want you to make positive changes in your life because it may change the way you relate to them. Delete the haters from your cell phone and your life.

DR. K: TURNING TORTURE INTO TREASURE

Fitting in movement had never been a challenge for me—I always found time and always tried new things. But during, and for some time after, the dark ages of breast cancer, movement was difficult because it was painful. However, with persistence, my function and energy did come back. I do not claim it was easy; it took a lot of self-motivation to stick to a schedule, to be patient, and to remind myself that true change takes time but does come with persistence. My dear friend would always remind me of his father's saying, "Persistent application toward one steadfast goal." Keep your eye on the prize, right? Thus, persistence became my new bestie, buddied-up to reach a destination—health and happiness!

I knew how to exercise, the movements. I knew how to develop a training program, but I found I needed motivation, which I hadn't needed before. I was a bit at a loss. But I really worked to enjoy movement again, just as I had in the past. I was surprised how much time it took to reduce the discomfort from incisions, from implants, from damage to tissues. But I just kept adding little bits of movement. I didn't overload with heavy resistance. I worked on improving range of motion and muscle endurance. And it came back, and so did my energy, and I felt like I was once again living in *my* body.

"You don't know what you've got until it's gone" is quite true. I hadn't realized just how important movement was to me until I couldn't move. However, in retrospect, maybe one isn't given more than one can handle. My experience taught me that movement is my passion and a gift I love to share with others. Experiencing the struggles of disease and rehabilitation taught me empathy, and now, working with my clients with movement limitations, I truly understand how tough it can be. The psychology of it all! How does one stay positive through a negative experience? And, health struggles can become very negative. You have to navigate through the health care system. You have to survive the ups and downs of rehabilitating. It's tough. But it can be done.

Little by little, I got stronger, I got faster, and I got happier. I had missed moving. It was my lost treasure, reclaimed. And that is what I have tried to teach my clients, including Chef D. And the MyTendWell Lifestyle Plan is the product we created to share the treasures of healthy movement and healthy food.

Join us on the MyTendWell journey!

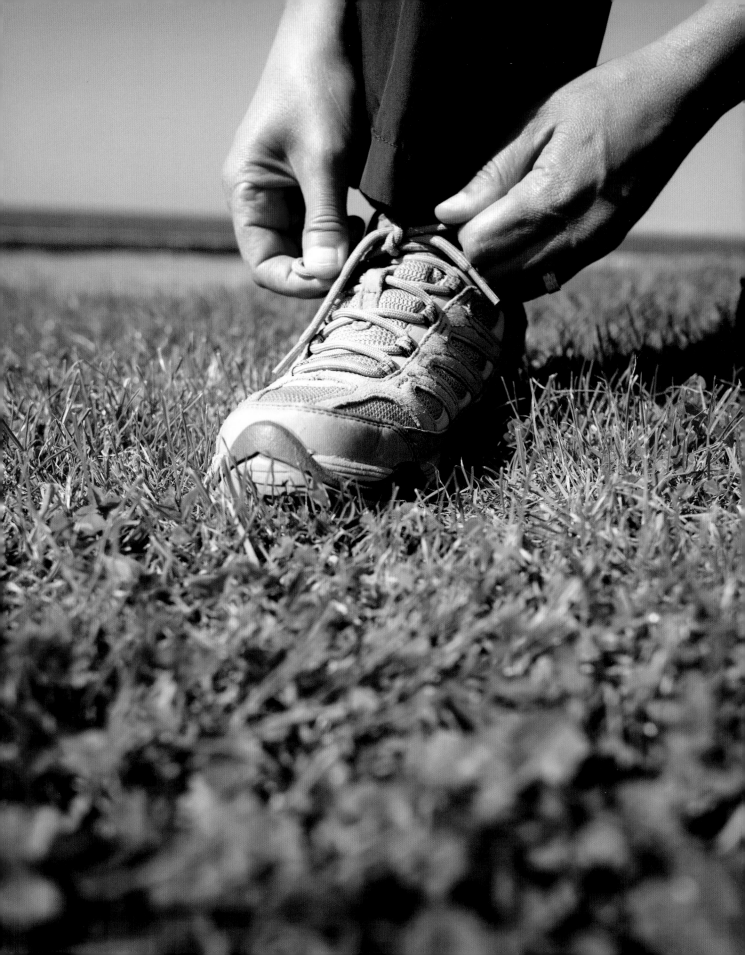

2 Who's Reading This Lifestyle Book?

STARTING IS THE HARDEST PART

Getting started is the hardest part of living a healthy lifestyle. Breaking patterns built over a lifetime ain't easy and many of us need help on this journey. Loved ones, friends, a trusted physician, or a good wellness coach are the most helpful. Sometimes family problems may have gotten you where you are in the first place, so, unless relations are truly supportive, you may want to rely on others or see a therapist. The first step is recognizing your desire to achieve a healthy lifestyle. By that I mean going ALL the way: finding your healthy body weight, changing your dietary choices, making time for daily exercise, and fulfilling your desire for longevity without disease. Once you decide to do it, you can really get going. But until you want it badly enough, it just won't stick. It has taken me about 40 years to figure this out, so take your time and be good to yourself. As RuPaul says, "If you don't love yourself, how the hell is anyone else gonna love you."

Think about it, there is nothing worse than being overweight and having trouble doing things that once were easy. For me it was having discomfort when bending down to tie my shoes. It was ridiculous. Only having a wardrobe of five outfits (all chef's clothes or sweatpants) became embarrassing, yet I still delayed getting started. To be honest, there was a lot of vanity involved with my getting back on the road to health. I didn't like the way I looked in pictures and felt uncomfortable at social events. I dreaded seeing people I hadn't seen for a while because I knew what "they'd be thinking." I didn't even look like the guy on the cover of my cookbooks. There are, of course, many other scarier reasons to live a healthier life, and seeing my father decline and die and my mother break her back all made things suddenly more clear. The time is now.

BEHAVIOR CHANGE

Changing behavior takes time, patience, and the ability to reflect and consider what may be helping and what may be hindering your progress. Consider the cognitive-behavioral process in figure 2.1 (continued in next textbox).

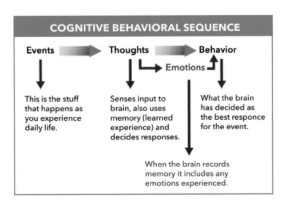

COGNITIVE BEHAVIORAL SEQUENCE

Events → Thoughts → Behavior
Emotions

This is the stuff that happens as you experience daily life.

Senses input to brain, also uses memory (learned experience) and decides responses.

What the brain has decided as the best responce for the event.

When the brain records memory it includes any emotions experienced.

WHAT MOTIVATES BEHAVIOR?

As you collect experiences, let's say through cooking, you learn motor skills and the value of having fun and working hard, among other things. These experiences become "mechanisms" such as motor programs, elation, and persistence, respectively. As learning continues, responses improve through capabilities such as efficiency (an elite-level swimmer is more efficient than a recreational swimmer), accuracy (an elite-level archer is more accurate than a novice), and even tenacity (elite-level performers dedicate the time and practice to achieve high-level performances). So, what motivates behavior? Enjoyment and interest in the activity help. But how do we get someone interested in physical activity? One thing that helps is to ask people what physical activities they find enjoyable. Chef D likes hiking and water exercise, and he sticks to it. Stay tuned for more on motivation.

STAGES OF CHANGE

How do you know if you are ready for change? Prochaska and DiClemente (1983) developed the Transtheoretical Model of Behavior Change (or Stages of Change), a psychological theory based on the idea that as people change behavior, they progress through distinct stages of change.

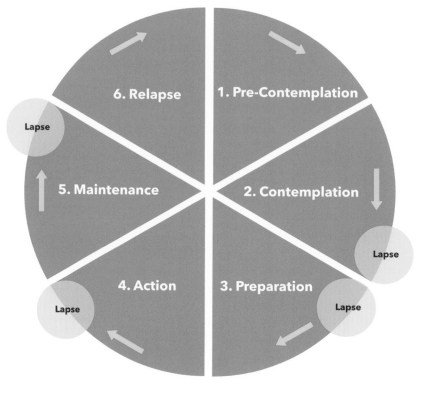

The Stages of Behavior

Precontemplation: No intent to change behavior within the foreseeable future (> 6 months)

Reasons: Uninformed

Demoralized

Defensive (against social pressure to change)

Applied to exercise-physical activity domain: Inactive and not considering exercise-physical activity

Contemplation: Serious intent to change within the next 6 months

May remain in this stage for up to two years: Chronic contemplators

Applied to exercise-physical activity domain: Inactive, considering starting exercise within 6 months

Preparation: Intend to take action within the near future (~1 month)

Have an action plan in mind

Applied to exercise-physical activity domain: Irregularly active but plan to start within 1 month

Action: Actively participating in new behavior within the past 6 months

This is the least stable stage

Applied to exercise-physical activity domain: Active for ≤ 6 months

Maintenance: Six months and longer after the criterion has been reached (i.e., regular exercise)

Applied to exercise-physical activity domain: Active for > 6 months

Termination: Five years of maintenance of the regular behavior (15-17% of ex-smokers and alcohol abusers)

Diet-related diseases include diabetes, heart disease, food allergies that can result in irritable bowel syndrome, diverticula in the colon, cancers of the stomach, colon, gallbladder, ovaries, or prostate, and lots of other yucky stuff. Not all of these are solely diet related, but studies have shown that "you are what you eat." And, ultimately, you do have control over what you put in your mouth. Prevention can be as simple as changing what you eat and going for a walk. It's learning that there is more to eating than just filling up. It's finding out that there is plenty of stuff that tastes great and isn't fried or overly processed with chemicals, preservatives, and colorings. It also means making physical activity something your life revolves around, not just a hassle you have to deal with because you are fat. Working out has to be a date you make with yourself, and loving yourself means you never break it without rescheduling it or without very good reason. The hardest part about exercise is that first step—like walking through the gym door. Once you've gotten that far, the rest is easy.

The first step in changing your eating habits is educating yourself about what you should be eating. Your body requires all components: (1) macronutrients: proteins, carbohydrates, and good fats; (2) micronutrients: vitamins and minerals (a diet that includes these nutrients has fruits, vegetables, lean meat, fish, and whole grains; and (3) phytonutrients: again it's fruits and vegetables. Having the desire to eat better is a start; actually beginning to eat better puts you on the road to better health. A 1 percent change is better than no change at all. Simply changing your diet can make the difference between feeling good and feeling tired. Food determines overweight or underweight bodies. Food will provide for a well-fueled body, or result in a nutrient-deficient one. Only you actually decide what you will put in your mouth. Choose wisely!

You just have to think that you are what you eat. Getting started happens when *you* want to achieve health by feeding your body the stuff

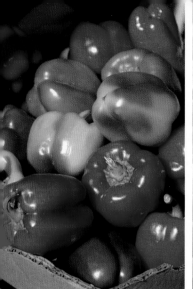
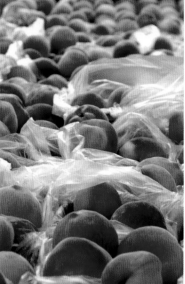
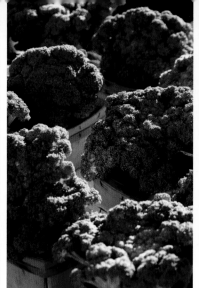
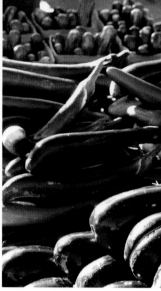

A colorful montage of produce contributes to nutritional wellness with these brilliant eggplant, peaches, peppers, and broccoli.

that will make it run like the ultimate power machine that it really is. I know it sounds simple and straightforward, but it is one of the toughest things there is to do. You'll find that once you've started, there is no turning back; your old lifestyle will no longer make sense. Once you make the change, you'll be asking yourself, "Why did I wait so long to get started?"

It is hard to know what information is correct—where to find valid information. Chef D and Dr. K are committed to teaching you the most current and accurate information about living a wellness lifestyle, and the first step is by teaching you the MyTendWell Lifestyle Plan's eight dimensions of wellness. But what is wellness? We see the word *wellness* all over the place—it takes on many meanings—from chiropractic offices to employee work clinics. So what is it? Broadly defined, it is living healthfully. But wellness is more than that; it is remaining free of disease, and it is having healthy relationships, with others and the environment. Wellness is like golf, always shooting for the better score. Wellness is progressing along a continuum toward optimal wellness. Always fine tuning and integrating the dimensions in order for you to reach total wellness. Chef D and Dr. K want you to learn how to live a wellness lifestyle and our plan teaches you the skills you need for a successful wellness lifestyle.

The MyTendWell Lifestyle Plan: *Eight Dimensions of Wellness*

Chef D and Dr. K's plan addresses eight dimensions of wellness and will teach you the pathways that move you along the continuum to optimal wellness.

Nutritional wellness requires awareness of current nutritional daily recommendations, such as eating whole grains, lean proteins, and a variety of fruits and vegetables every day.

Physical wellness is the persistent and deliberate effort to achieve and maintain your optimum level of physical activity and to assure good self-care through preventive medical exams. Achieving physical wellness consists of finding programs and activities that stimulate interest as well as address health-related concerns, such as low-back pain or cardiovascular functioning. Chef D and Dr. K encourage everyone to discuss their health with their physician prior to beginning an exercise program. Chef D and Dr. K also stress the importance of learning about your body and your health through Chef D and Dr. K's MyTendWell Lifestyle Plan. The plan provides information on functional and corrective exercise movements as well as encourages individuals to seek out fun recreational activities such as hiking, biking, kayaking, and gardening, to name a few.

Self-love and motivation are two important components of behavior change

Self-love, rather the cognition and perception of self, are psychological (and sociological) theories or concepts/constructs that describe individual feelings, ideas, and beliefs of self. Not easy concepts to describe in a textbox, but I like a challenge. How we feel or think of ourselves is instrumental to how we behave. Revolutionary, I know. But follow along, please. I will make my point. For example, if you perceive yourself as successful within a specific context, say a sport, then you are more likely to seek out opportunities to participate. Subsequent participation (deliberate practice over time) within that context will enhance your learning and thus improve your skills. Improvement in skills will enhance your success, which will in turn boost your confidence, especially within that context. Your confidence increases as a result of your *competence*—simply put, when we are successful, we feel competent. This confidence will then enhance self-efficacy. *Self-efficacy* is belief in your ability to be successful in a specific behavior. Thus, as you become more successful, self-efficacy increases. This in turn modifies how you perceive and think of yourself, affecting your identity and self-concept positively—to Chef D, this is self-love: having a positive view of self, and knowing you are competent.

Competence implies mastery of a skill. Watch Chef D in the kitchen and you'll see it for yourself. Chef D's mastery of culinary arts reinforces his going into the kitchen. Essentially his success enhances his desire to continue to create new dishes, to develop new business practices, and to tend to his guests. All of these skills were developed; and the pursuit to develop these skills required time and deliberate practice.

Anders Erickson identified that it takes about 10,000 hours of deliberate practice to achieve elite-level performance. But what is it that *motivates* practice? Why would someone spend 10,000 hours practicing something? That is the critical question. Chef D *liked* cooking as a kid. He was recognized early on and appeared in his hometown newspaper for his culinary skills. Because he liked to cook, he sought out opportunities to cook. He worked (i.e., deliberate practice) with local chefs and was *supported* and encouraged by his family, especially his mom—who continues to support him.

So, two important things: liking something and support of this interest. Remember these. We are coming back to them.

The critical question is, what *motivates* someone to practice?

There are two forms of motivation, *intrinsic* and *extrinsic*.

Intrinsic motivation is what's inside, so to speak, such as enjoyment and competence (sound familiar?), and demonstrated through behaviors such as interest and desire to participate in an activity. Importantly, intrinsic motivation is key to someone sticking with an activity or behavior.

Extrinsic motivation is the stuff on the outside, such as praise and medals. However, these things are less important in contributing to someone sticking to an activity or behavior, whereas participation due to extrinsic factors, such as enjoyment, have a more persistent effect.

So back to Chef D. He has always been motivated to cook and to learn new ways to cook. But motivation to cook doesn't motivate him to exercise. How then does Chef D find motivation to start exercising? Stay tuned! (More in chap. 3.)

Social wellness means balancing and integrating yourself with friends and family as well as with other individuals you encounter in life such as coworkers and community members. Social wellness includes supporting and participating in community events. Chef D and Dr. K encourage individuals to find opportunities to enhance social wellness. We will provide suggestions.

Emotional wellness is made up of your attitudes and beliefs toward self and toward life. This includes having a positive and realistic self-concept, self-identity, and self-esteem. Emotional wellness also pertains to the awareness and the control of feelings and your ability to act autonomously to cope with stress while maintaining fulfilling relationships with others.

Environmental wellness involves a balance between home and work life, and the reciprocal relationship between you and your environment (nature, community). Achieving environmental wellness necessitates your evaluation of the environment in which you live, work, and play, and perhaps the redesigning of that environment to be more conducive and supportive to an active life. You will need to assess your work environment to determine if the interface between you and your workstation is ideal and promotes a healthy musculoskeletal system.

Intellectual wellness involves stimulating yourself intellectually by learning new skills through reading to enhancing cognitive functioning. Cognitive functioning is a big topic. Researchers are constantly looking for the answers to what improves or maintains cognitive functioning. Pleasingly, many investigations of cognitive functioning are demonstrating that, in addition to reading, playing cards, and word and math games, physical activity also impacts cognitive functioning in a positive way. The MyTendWell Lifestyle Plan encourages you to *work out* your cognitive functioning through mental and physical stimulation. Knowledge *is* power.

Spiritual wellness is having a positive perception of meaning and purpose in life, as well as recognition and acceptance of a unifying and integrating force between mind and body. Chef D and Dr. K encourage individuals to spend time on spiritual wellness. This can be time spent reviewing your day, and/or your life, through reflection, and by using tools such as meditation, relaxation, group chats, and prayer.

Occupational wellness depends on one's attitude toward work and feelings of satisfaction from work. Importantly, occupational wellness also considers leisure time, or time away from work. Occupational wellness is the balance of work and play. MyTendWell knows that all work and no play make for a dull flower, so Chef D and Dr. K educate you about the best practices for occupational wellness. Dr. K's background includes ergonomics and workplace wellness and she teaches you how to evaluate your workplace and how best to fit your job to you, and you to your job.

Tips for Nutritional Wellness

We incur one of our biggest expenses buying groceries, with the average family's weekly spending ranging between $150 and $300. Chef D and Dr. K provide some great tips for growing and preserving your own food to assist in lowering food expenses as well as in really knowing what you are eating.

Keeping fresh foods fresh is not easy; Chef D and Dr. K provide some great tips for food freshness.

Chef D's Quick Tip: Keep washed lettuces and greens crisp and garden-fresh by placing stem ends in a tall container with just enough water to keep the stems submerged. Keep this container in the fridge—your lettuces and greens will last longer.

Tips for Physical Wellness

If there is a "magic pill" that improves health, it *is* physical activity. Physical activity and

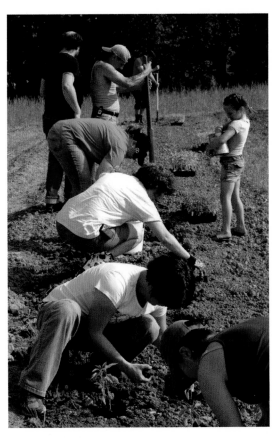

Many hands make light work for the FARMhands staff in their community garden all while working toward three dimensions of wellness: environmental, social, and physical.

exercise provide benefits for many health concerns.

High blood glucose levels can contribute to diabetes. Pricelessly, physical activity can reduce blood glucose levels. By the year 2050, one in three people will have type 2 diabetes (a completely preventable disease).

Enhancing general mood is a sWell thing! And that magic pill has been demonstrated to improve mood in one single bout of exercise.

Dr. K's Quick Tip: Invite your friends for a "Hike with Those I Like." Find a local park or wildlife refuge and pick a trail to spend time hiking with friends while enjoying the outdoors. Keep your eyes peeled for wildlife, keep

your posture in check, and be sure to keep good footing. This one activity will address multiple MyTendWell dimensions: physical (hiking), social (friends), outdoors (environmental).

Dr. K's Daily Must Do Item: Move.

Tips for Social Wellness

Time spent with friends and family, enjoying each other and enjoying the moment, can be a huge boost to mood and relationships.

Chef D's Quick Tip: Chef D, an expert in social events, is an excellent host to his guests. You leave his table feeling cared for and lifted up. Dr. K challenges you to invite your friends for a unique social outing. My friends and clients own a large nursery and garden center and have recently been offering events such as a workshop for learning to build a succulent planter. These have been so successful and are great opportunities for groups of friends to get together (social wellness), learn a new skill (intellectual wellness), and make a green space (environmental wellness). See, one little outing addresses at least three dimensions of wellness. And you are supporting a local business. Share your wellness (go to www.mytendwell.com to share your wellness).

Chef D and Dr. K's Daily Must Do Item: Share a smile!

Tips for Emotional Wellness

Having a positive view of yourself is important. Past successes and past failures contribute to your perspective, or perception, of self. It was important to address this dimension early on when Chef D and I began working together on his wellness plan. Chef D spells this out in his journey in chapter 1. So he has been working on his perception of self—what he calls **self-love**.

Quick Tip: Create short-term, achievable goals that will assist in building your confidence and ultimately your self-efficacy, which will enhance your emotional wellness and overall wellness.

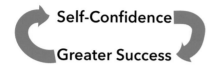

Self-Confidence

Greater Success

Tips for Spiritual Wellness

Spirituality has its meaning for each of us. What is important is we practice good spiritual wellness. Find a spiritual path that is yours. Research that discipline or practice and find ways to interact with others who share your beliefs.

Chef D's Quick Tip: Visit places that evoke spiritual connections. I was just watching *CBS Sunday Morning* and a segment on Last Stand Hill in Montana (Custer's Last Stand), and the National Park Guide described the place as "spiritual." Find places that are spiritual for you.

Tips for Occupational Wellness

Sedentary behavior is a risk factor for many health-related issues, including musculoskeletal concerns such as low-back pain and obesity. Dr. K provides solutions for decreasing sedentary behavior, especially while at work.

Dr. K's Quick Tip: Dr. K suggests taking *station breaks* every two hours during prolonged sitting tasks such as working at a computer workstation. Prolonged sitting contributes to poor health, from metabolic to musculoskeletal. Getting up and performing deliberate movement every two hours will improve muscle health, stimulate your brain, and generally

wake up your body. Dr. K prescribes walking around office space, hallways, or stairways, and, if possible, getting outdoors and perhaps walking around the building. Performing corrective exercises assists in correcting poor posture and working muscles that need to be worked.

MyTendWell CHALLENGE

The ties that bind a community are vital for future success. Dr. K does live in a small town and small towns are threatened just as some animals are. Loss of industry and changes in agricultural practices have jeopardized rural communities and excluded them from the global game. A small community in central Illinois has found another way to keep a community alive. Casey, Illinois, is home to the biggest rocking chair, pitchfork, knitting needles, wind chimes, and more. Local residents thought outside the box to create revenue. One local resident, Jim Bolin, decided to build the world's largest wind chimes to draw visitors to the town. It worked and the idea grew. Pardon the pun. Casey now has a tourism industry. People flock to see the world record holding items. Mr. Bolin's dream to keep his small hometown alive is a perfect example of environmental and social wellness.

Chef D and Dr. K challenge you to get involved in your community. Volunteer with community cleanup, coach a little league team, or start a community garden.

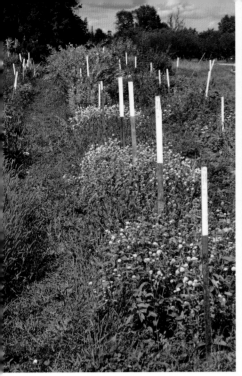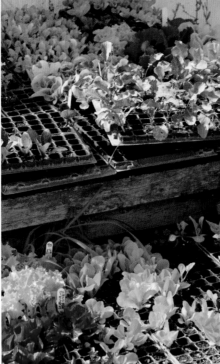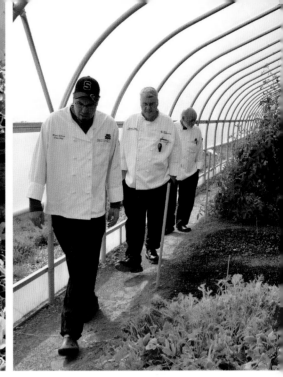

Student Organic Farms at Michigan State is a template for you to create your own community garden and compete in the MyTendWell Community Wellness Challenge.

Tips for Environmental Wellness

Our environments provide our resources for living. We grow our foods—grains, fruits, and vegetables—as well as raise or harvest our meats and fish. Unfortunately, not all food production, from harvest to table, uses sustainable methods. MyTendWell wants to help educate individuals about sustainable practices.

Food packaging is just one source of waste that piles up in our landfills each day. Items such as packaging materials, organic compounds, and other recyclables, such as aluminum, mound up in landfills each year.

The US population, about 5 percent of the world population, is the #1 trash-producing country in the world, generating over 1,600 pounds per person each year, equaling 40 percent of the world's garbage. MyTendWell wants to inform more individuals about better environmental practices.

Quick Tip: Reduce, Reuse, and Recycle.

Reduce: Buy local foods that aren't packaged in boxes.

Reuse: Try your hand at home canning and preserve some of those seasonal treats. Canning vegetables in reusable Mason jars cuts down on the number of cans and bags we throw out. You are also canning those yummy, fresh organic veggies you grew or bought from a local farmer or farmers' market.

Recycle: Find out what materials your community recycles and utilize that facility to the best of your ability.

Tips for Intellectual Wellness

Lifelong learning is a requirement to continue to move along the wellness continuum. New research is always out there—new trends and new gadgets and new technology. It's work to just stay up to date. MyTendWell works to consolidate information on wellness (visit **www.mytendwell.com** for news in wellness).

Quick Tip: Keep doing what you are doing. You bought or borrowed this book; you are seeking out information. You want to learn, too. Read on!

STARTING THE MyTendWell LIFESTYLE PLAN: FIVE STEPS TO WELLNESS

Step 1: Identify where you are within Prochaska and DiClemente's Model of Stages of Change.

Step 2: Write out your SMART Goals (chapter 3).

Step 3: Start recording daily entries for 30 days (minimum) in your log (chapter 3).

Step 4: Assemble your Toolbox and your Pantry (chapter 3).

Step 5: Schedule your physical activity like an appointment and plan your meals for the week ahead.

Now do it!

mytendwell.com

THE BASICS IN THE PROVERBIAL NUTSHELL: REGIME CUISINE BASICS

By sticking to the program of preparing fresh, organic food simply, reducing portions, increasing plant foods and fiber, reducing consumption of meat and saturated fat, and moving your body regularly, we all can attain and maintain a higher level of health and experience a higher quality of life. Here are your special MyTendWell Lifestyle Plan guidelines:

- Balancing protein, carbohydrate, and healthy fats (see tables 5.1 and 5.2)

- Eating more organic and naturally produced foods and sea vegetables (seaweeds, most of which may be found in Asian markets)

- Consuming more complex carbohydrates and fewer refined carbohydrates such as white bread, muffins, crackers, and bagels

- Consuming more fruits, vegetables, fiber, legumes, and whole grains

- Reducing consumption of sweets, sugars, carbonated beverages, juices, and caffeine

- Consuming more fish high in omega-3 fatty acids, lean meats, and eliminating meat processed with hormones

- Consuming more grass-fed, less grain-fed, meat products

- Eliminating processed foods with additives and coloring agents

- Reducing and eliminating snack foods, frozen prepared meals, and many canned foods. But remember, some frozen and canned vegetables can be more nutritious than improperly processed and shipped fresh vegetables.

- Reducing intake of saturated fats and increasing intake of unsaturated fats; eliminating consumption of trans and hydrogenated fats

- Decreasing portion sizes

- Reducing hard alcohol intake

- Daily movement (exercise, physical activity) for your body. Just Move!

- Drinking 32 to 48 ounces of water per day

- Sharing in food preparation and enjoyment of food, wine, and pleasures of the table

- Balancing rest and work

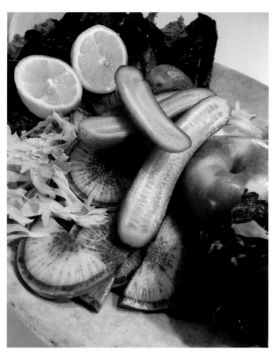

A cornucopia of fruits and veggies feeds the eyes and the body.

WHY WE OVEREAT

There is a vast multitude of reasons for overeating; some reasons are baffling and some are actually crippling. The popular image of the overweight mother taunting her children to make sure they finish what's on their plates is one very good reason. Another reason is the barrage of advertisements grabbing attention on the television no matter what time of day. Larger portion sizes in the home and especially in fast-food restaurants contribute to overeating. Depression, anxiety, stress, and numerous other physiological, psychological, and cultural factors play roles in why people overeat. For me there is a very personal battle that involves comfort, escape, and fear.

In my life I've been both incredibly healthy and terribly out shape . . . several times, flip-flopping from one to the other and never understanding why I was having such unhappiness with crafting my self-image, while other people, on either side of the spectrum, seem to just go along so easily. It took 9/11 to really get me down again. And for the year that followed, I ate my way to an all-time high, scale-tilting level. I guess the sadness hit me so deeply that I couldn't deal with it, and to avoid that feeling, I ate all the things I normally was careful to limit. I ate them until I filled the void of the loss I was feeling. And I worked long, long hours. It didn't take much time until I felt the weight gain hitting me, and I stopped going to the gym and exercising outdoors because I felt embarrassed about my appearance. You would think I'd try to change when I saw this happening, but I didn't. All I wanted to do was not feel.

As we overeat, our stomachs become accustomed to a certain amount of food, and our bodies end up storing the excess calories as fat. This is a vicious cycle that psychologically is difficult to break. We get used to eating a certain amount of food and will not feel satiated without that fullness. Overeating can lead to obesity, which in turn can lead to more serious health problems, such as high blood pressure, cardiovasvcular disease, and type 2 diabetes. I truly love food and

MAKE TIME FOR PLAY

All work and no play makes Jack a dull boy! The old sayings we are all familiar with aren't usually far from the truth. Too much work dulls our health, and lack of play steals our happiness. In fact, the repeated activation of the HPA (hypothalamus-pituitary-adrenal) axis, specifically the secretion of cortisol from the adrenal glands without adequate rest and recovery, causes overexposure to this stress hormone. This can lead to health issues such as weight gain and decreased immune functioning. So save some time for play.

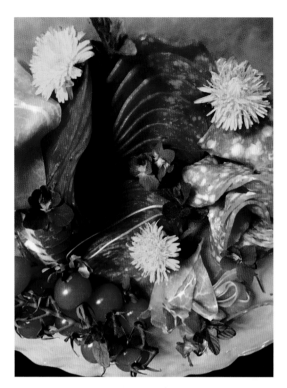
Meat sweats platter.

Paleolithic man possibly spent many hours and perhaps days without large quantities of food. Instead, grazing on roots, tubers, seeds, and nuts helped to stave off hunger and keep fat reserves in check. When meat, most likely not the main food source, was available, all parts of the animal were eaten. And the family, or in those days, the group, was satisfied. Hunger was probably an accepted part of life, and available

cooking and give high priority to the adventure found in partaking and experiencing as much of what is out there as possible. I love to share food and wine with family and friends and can't have too many dinner and cocktail parties. What a contradictory life I was leading, a true love-hate relationship! For a chef, food is always available. At the restaurant we make some damn good French fries; hand cut and cooked twice in peanut oil. The first time is to cook them through in lower heated fat, the second is to send them on a high-heat trip to crispness. They topped my list on mindless snacking. They're so hard to turn down . . . I didn't. I did think about eating "healthy" during those days and would often skip meals instead of eating something bad. But at night, after a cocktail or three, nothing was out of bounds. Often I'd sit on the couch with my twin tuxedo kittens and fill my face with carbs, sharing time not with real people but with whatever late-night host was on Comedy Central. It was comfortable.

WHY EATING BECOMES DISORDERED

Why do we fall into negative relationships with food? The need to control something? The desire to achieve an ideal weight? Stress? Depression? Not enough time to prepare and enjoy a meal? All can negatively affect eating behaviors. Food can be a source of comfort and enjoyment; food can quickly be used to change moods by activating the same reward circuits as some drugs. Foods stimulate the hedonic system (pleasure/reward) and evidence is suggesting that refined sugars and processed foods have a similar, albeit weaker, effect on the brain as opioids do.

Binge eaters typically eat energy-rich foods such as breads and pastas as well as sugary, high-fat, and salty snack foods. Food marketers are well aware of the human brain's response to these foods. Creative and influential marketing, a stressful world, and perhaps some self-doubt make the perfect storm for overeating. What's the best-intentioned but sugar-crazed brain to do to beat the binge? (See the upcoming Top Five Tips to Avoid Overeating.)

WHEN EATING BECOMES DISORDERED

Chef D and Dr. K both experience some disordered eating. For me, I often work with clients or teach classes during mealtimes—breakfast, lunch, and dinner—so I end up eating on an "alternative" schedule. It is not uncommon for me to hit the kitchen, starving from a busy day; it becomes a grab and gobble fest. This is not a good eating practice. I eat all those things the brain craves, breads, chips—empty calories that don't feed my body but just satisfy cravings. The solution for me is to prepare meals ahead of time. If I don't, I will end up feeling run-down with low energy, and no one wants a draggy wellness coach.

Chef D was a late-night snacker. He would skip breakfast and just have a cup of black coffee. He would then graze his way through his workday—not eating a real meal until after 7:00 p.m. He found himself hungry again at 11:00 p.m. and grabbed whatever was in the pantry or deep freezer.

food was cherished. Have you actually ever been truly hungry? We all say, "I'm starving," but are you really? As a chef and a citizen of the culinary world, I, too, am constantly searching for food but to satisfy a very different longing. As a chef I'm also searching to bring happiness to others by creating dishes to excite and amaze. And for myself, I was searching for an end to the sadness and pain that crept into my brain. I used food as a Band-Aid that made it all feel better.

In the United States, and most developed countries, so much food is available at any time of day that most people never really get hungry. Eating three large meals a day on top of snack foods really adds up the calories. We wouldn't overeat if we spent more time outdoors, away from the television that force-feeds food advertisements. We probably wouldn't overeat if we thought that we may not have food tomorrow and we should savor, in small amounts, what we have today. Just because food is available 24 hours a day doesn't mean we must eat it. This is a difficult concept for many people to understand. Food should be wholesome, pleasurable, nourishing, healthy, and, above all, not in excess. I should understand this more than most folks. My first book was filled with healthy, great-tasting recipes, yet I had lost the will to follow them. The past seemed so far gone and the future so

BEATING THE BINGE: TOP FIVE TIPS TO AVOID OVEREATING

1. Have a game plan—plan your meals for the week. Shop ahead and prepare salads and other make-ahead dishes that will then be ready for you.

2. Write down your meals on your MyTendWell journal. Be sure to include why you did or didn't eat and any feelings or emotions associated with the meal.

3. Drink a large glass of water before eating.

4. Eliminate access to your trigger foods. Don't have them in the house, or keep them out of sight as best as you can.

5. Keep healthy snacks available—make a fruit/veggie "party" tray and keep the party at home.

unsure. I questioned if it was worth the energy and time to get myself back together. Well, we know the answer. Of course it is! I've found that one of the hardest things to do is to put my arms around myself to give me the hug I need and the kind of respectful love we can only give ourselves. In times of trouble or insecurity we tend to worry about the ones around us. It is so much easier to take care of others because we know they need it. Our own needs are put aside until we find the desire to look inward once again and to look outward with hope.

HEY MAN, TAKE A WALK ON THE WILD SIDE

We've talked about food, now let's talk about drink.

The image of a cocaine-tooting, pot-smoking, booze-guzzling rock star chef is not far off point. When I was living the New York City celebrity chef lifestyle I did about everything there was out there to do. Night club ropes dropped for me and my chef friends. Rounds of drinks and free snacks arrived out of nowhere at the trendy downtown industry after-hour joints. Free tasting menus and alcohol pairings were offered at the best restaurants across the city. Artists and musicians who came to the restaurant invited me to gallery openings and concerts and actors gave me tickets to their theater openings and television shows. We even did "after parties" at Guastavinos for *SNL* and *Sex in the City*. Mick Jagger, Madonna, Prince (he may have been known as a symbol at that time), Beyoncé (Destiny's Child back then), and Aerosmith were in and out of the dining rooms of the restaurants I worked. It was the time of my life . . . at that time of my life. I never knew exactly what was going to happen after I left the restaurant, but I knew I wasn't going to go straight home!

I did think about my health, well, as much as a young guy in Manhattan does. I was a gym bunny and Rollerbladed everywhere. Even with

bags of produce from the Union Square Market back to La Grenouille on 52nd street. But back then it was all about vanity and ego. I wanted to look good; I knew I could always find something else to make me feel good. It was New York City after all. You had "a guy" for everything you needed. And I'm not just talking about dry cleaning . . .

Lots of people say they work hard and play hard. But chefs really talk the talk and walk the walk. Many chefs get stuck in the pattern of their glory days, and it swallows them up. I've seen many a career (even lives) shortened by the excesses of booze, pills, smoke, coke, dope, and cigarettes—combos not for the faint of heart but perfect for a young man with too much money and no responsibilities, except to his restaurant and his crew. The ones that do get away unscathed usually are snatched up by a strong man or woman; angels who are in love with them despite their bad behavior, pulling them kicking and screaming to a more "normal" and sustainable lifestyle. The guys in the biz often are saved with a wedding ring or fatherhood, though often not in that order.

In my 50s and still childless and single, I luckily dodged the bullet of addiction. I've been close at times but have managed to escape the talons of that chasing dragon. Back then I kept my recreational drugs for the weekends (Sundays and Mondays), never feeling controlled by them. Booze on the other hand, especially wine, is a love affair that stole my heart. Wine and beer go so well with food that it's hard to say no. Champagne with your eggs Benedict? S'il vous plaît. A draft beer with fish and chips at lunch? Yes, please. A good zin with my venison "roti" and celery root gratin? Absolutely! After moving back to the Midwest I discovered a love for bourbon, and that, too, is a tricky mistress . . . so sexy and smooth, but able to turn around and kick your ass.

If you feel that booze or drugs are controlling you, find a friend or family member and figure out the best way to get help. If you want to cut down on alcohol but don't want to give it up completely, here are some clues to keeping your favorite dinner companion a friend without it becoming an enemy. Who knows, you might even find that life without it is even more enjoyable.

BOOZE CLUES

- Drink lots of water before a meal being served with alcohol, and drink one glass of water per alcoholic drink during the evening.

- Find new ways to "reward" yourself for a hard day's work or rigorous workout or sporting event.

- Don't replace food calories with alcohol calories. Eat good high fiber, low glycemic meals throughout the day and enjoy alcohol as a separate social event accompanied by food.

- Cut back on sweets at the same time you cut alcohol. They react somewhat in the same way in the body as alcohol and you might crave them, too.

- Shake up your schedule. Start new habits and drop some old ones, and make sure you are consistent with both.

- Restructure your free time: think of things you really love and miss doing and do them.

- Make homemade nonalcoholic beverages like Kvass, Kambuchi tea, and drinkable vinegars that are full of beneficial probiotics. This makes a great hobby and is something you can share with others. They are surprisingly satisfying replacements.

- Try incorporating unsweetened fruit juices like unsweetened cranberry and tart cherry instead of wine with dinner. They look the same

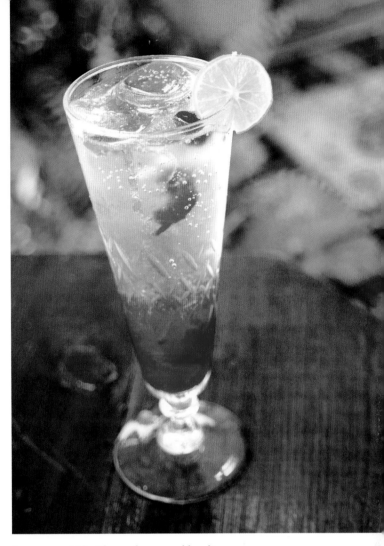

Agave aperitif with cranberry and key lime.

in your glass and pair with food well. Plus they are great for you.

- Create a new "cocktail hour" by sharing fun and beautiful nonalcoholic drinks with family and friends. This is a fun time to use fresh or unsweetened fruit juices and mix them with sparkling water or tonic. Bring out your collection of flavored bitters and have fun with garnishes like starfruit, fresh cranberries, citrus, fruit, vegetables, and herbs.

- At brunch, come up with nonalcoholic riffs on Bloody Marys and mimosas that are as impressive to look at as they are fun to drink.

TRIGGERS

What makes you put a gun to your head . . . or a doughnut in your mouth?

Let's start by saying Sigmund Freud was right! All your problems are because of your mother. . . . Just kidding, MOM! But seriously, they are. After all, if she hadn't given birth to you, you wouldn't have any problems. But now you are an adult, and you have to take responsibility for your life and actions. It is hard to break old patterns that have allowed our inner child to have control of our adult bodies. There are lots of educated professionals who can help you talk it out, and it is worth the time and money to speak to a therapist if you feel you need assistance. But, if you feel fairly stable and want to go it alone, you need to start by figuring out what your triggers are.

"DIET stands for Did I Eat That?"—Unknown

What makes you mad, sad, happy, depressed, mentally or physically tired, hungry, and thirsty? What makes you laugh, cry, or reach for a Twinkie, a greasy burger, a soda, or a cocktail? Now that we are of an age when we should know better, what makes you act like an infant again? Craving comfort and security is natural, but it isn't appropriate if you are doing damage to yourself or to those around you. The first step in creating the lifestyle you want to lead is to figure out what you want and what is keeping you from getting it. These are usually feelings and thoughts that trigger us into falling into patterns that we have grown out of in our daily lives and that return to drag us back, kicking and screaming, to behaviors we regret. You are your leader; only you and your brain can make the changes needed to achieve successful long-term changes.

For me, these have been many different things at many different times. I was insecure about my sexuality from the age of 10 and felt I needed to keep it hidden. I was more of an artistic kid and loved crafts, gardening, cooking (of course), and other left-brained creative endeavors. Sports were never my strong suit, but I felt I wasn't a good son if I didn't succeed at them. I lost a brother at the age of 10 and that changed the complete dynamics of our family. When I was a young and upcoming chef I craved the limelight and was jealous of others who had reached it before me. I have been jealous of my brother for the traditional family he has built while I remain forever single. Running a restaurant is a huge challenge day in and day out. It is definitely not for the faint of heart. In addition, love affairs and breakups, deaths of grandparents, friends, employees, and parents all have enormous effects on our human brains. Something has to give! That is where most of us pull the trigger and regress into comfortable, nostalgic, and unhealthy ways of childhood thinking and youthful habits that we know better than to repeat. Mental stress and discomfort in our bodies are also triggers. Uncomfortable work and social interactions or being totally pooped at the end of a long day can allow us to fall back into the warm arms of our egos, where we are promised the old pleasures of unhealthy behaviors.

WHY ARE WE TOXIC?

There are lots of things that contribute to our toxic bodies, from internal stress to environmental contaminants. Regardless of the source, toxins contribute to disease and premature death. The evidence is clear that environmental exposure to toxins is prevalent and the relative risk to human health is discernable. But what can we do to decrease the risk? First and foremost, reduce environmental contamination. Organic agricultural processes can reduce the buildup of toxins in soils and water systems as well as the

HOW LONG DO TOXINS STICK AROUND?

How long a substance stays in the body or the soil and water depends on what type of chemical compound it is.

Lead: half-life in the bones of 20–30 years

Mercury: half-life in the blood of 57 days

Glyphosate: half-life in soil up to 22 years

contamination of food products either by direct application (pesticide residues on vegetables and fruits) or by the buildup of toxins in animal products from consumption of toxins in grains and water. Second, detoxification methods, such as cleanses through food and drink,

THE EFFECTS OF ENVIRONMENTAL CONTAMINANTS

- reproductive disorders such as infertility, birth defects, and perinatal mortality

- neurobehavioral disorders

- Parkinson's disease

- neurological disorders

- cognitive and psychomotor dysfunction

- cancer, including breast, endometrium, prostate, ovarian, thyroid, bone, testes, skin, and brain

are becoming much more common and may be beneficial in decreasing toxic contaminants.

Contamination stemming from environmental exposures to toxins has increased due to the increased use of pesticides and herbicides in lawn care application and agricultural practices. Spillage and leakage of chemicals and heavy metals from landfills, drift, and runoff from the agrochemical applications are all sources of contamination that do not stop at the edge of the field or golf course. Rather, it seeps into the soil, flows down the waterways, is carried on the wind, and clings to the very produce it was developed to increase the yield of or to the greens and fairways it was developed to make look pristine. The public needs to be made aware that these many contaminants, which were designed to withstand time and the elements and to destroy pests and plant life, are not easily degraded and hang around for a long time, adding to our opportunity for exposure.

Caveat Emptor!

Where does your food come from? You need to be informed about the growing and production practices of the foods you are eating and preparing for your family and friends. Chef D and Dr. K accentuate the use of organic food products. Food contamination from the use of agrochemicals in commercial farming is concerning for our health, and especially our children's health. Toxicity from substances such as agrochemicals, home-cleaning chemicals, air particulates, water pollutants, and so on, is an exposure problem. The more exposure, the higher the risk of a problem becomes. Thus, today's young ones are at risk of increased exposure because of the increased use of chemicals. For instance, do you hire a lawn care company to spray your yard? I have neighbors who are on the annual plan—four applications per year—one in spring, two in summer, and one in fall. Do without perfect lawns! The runoff as well as the particulates you are tracking into your home contribute to your exposure. Research investigations suggest

DID YOU KNOW OUR KIDS ARE AT GREATER RISK?

Exposure has a cumulative effect, just as the chemotherapy (remember, poison?) I received during breast cancer treatment had a cumulative effect; that is, the farther along in treatment you get, the more accentuated the side effects become (i.e., with the first dose you feel bad, but by the fourth dose you feel really bad). The chemo builds up in your body; the more there is, the greater the effect. This is the same with environmental contaminants that we are exposed to. Our kids have potentially been exposed since they were in utero, depending on what their moms have been exposed to. Further, the nature of infants and children to play indoors and outdoors and place toys and hands in their mouths, in addition to their higher metabolic rates and need for more calories, places them at greater risk of exposure. Because of their closer proximity to the ground, infants and children are more likely to come into contact with agrochemicals either by direct tactile contact or by inhalation of particulate matter within the air.

agrochemical contamination is prevalent and is associated with many acute and chronic health conditions, from asthma to cancer.

Stress

Stress is bad for our bodies. Stress is stress, regardless of the trigger, and the body has (among others) a response—cortisol! Yes, you've heard of it. You've probably rubbed cortisol cream (hydrocortisone) on an itchy spot. Well, our bodies, to be specific our adrenal glands, secrete

glucocorticoids in response to any stressful trigger or situation. There is evidence suggesting that prolonged exposure to cortisol has negative consequences and may contribute to health problems such as

- increased storage of body fat— weight gain!

- increased resistance to insulin—diabetes!

- decreased immune functioning, leading to an increase in illness and disease

- fatigue

- muscle loss

- ulcers

- infertility

- accelerated degeneration of neural structures and functioning

- depression

Depression

Depression results in a loss of interest or pleasure in activities, changes in sleep and/or appetite, feelings of guilt, hopelessness, sadness, difficulty making decisions, and/or fatigue, to list some symptoms. These symptoms occur nearly daily, all day. Depression ranks fourth in disability and early death. Treatment for depression ranges from medications to therapy; however, exercise has also been found to be effective in improving mood. Some treatments include a combination of medications, therapy, and exercise. What is important is that even one single bout of exercise has demonstrated positive improvements in mood.

Smoking

What is the leading preventable cause of death in the United States? Yep, smoking, and, no, you don't win a cigar.

Smoking contributes to the onset of numerous diseases, from cardiovascular diseases to cancers. In fact, if smoking were eliminated, one of every three cancer-related deaths would not occur. The statistics on smoking are expansive and conclusive—it's bad for you. Don't smoke, and encourage others to quit, too. (For more information on smoking, visit **www.cdc.gov/tobacco**.)

Texting and Driving

Far too often, I am driving and I see another driver texting, either reading or sending a text. This is STUPID! It is NOT possible to perform these two tasks (dual tasking) simultaneously at 100 percent efficiency for each task.

My PhD is in Motor Control and Learning, the area of study interested in topics such as attention. An early definition is "focalization, concentration. It implies withdrawal from some things in order to deal effectively with others" (James 1890). Think of attention as a fixed capacity for processing information. As that capacity is exceeded (think overload), performance (of a task) will degrade. More straightforwardly put, no one can perform two tasks (texting and driving) at 100 percent. The attentional demand of performing one task detracts from the performance of the other task.

Mythbuster: "I'm a good multitasker!" Chef D and Dr. K debate this. Chef D thinks simmering a stew and arranging flowers is good multitasking, when, in fact, he is just organizing his activities. Multitasking is attempting to execute two tasks simultaneously.

DISTRACTED DRIVING

This is any activity that distracts the driver's attention from the primary task–driving! This includes talking to others in the car, surfing the radio for channels, and eating.

The consequences: 3,477 people were killed and 391,000 were injured from distracted drivers in 2015. (For more information on distracted driving visit NHTSA at www.nhtsa.gov.)

THE EVIL EMPIRE–SLAYING THE ARCHENEMIES IN YOUR PANTRY

When I was growing up in southern Indiana I would jump off the school bus and run to the basement, usually with a bag of chips, pretzels, or popcorn (Chef D's Mom doesn't recall having "bags of chips" in their home) to watch reruns of *The Lone Ranger*. Good and evil were literally spelled out in black and white. Later, for the next generation of school children, the same scenario played out again in the *Star Wars* series with Luke against Darth and his dark evil empire.

"Why do people keep their scales in the bathroom? They should keep them in the kitchen. I think I'd feel guilty eating a bag of Oreos if I knew the scale was watching me." —Unknown

Well, in a healthy kitchen we need to forget about all that. Color wise, it is the exact opposite that represents evil. When you see white, you need to be frightened. The dark whole grains and leafy green vegetables are the superheroes (see the Tremendous 20 in chap. 4), and the white flour, white sugar, and refined white starches are the bad guys. That's what I call "white trash." They are all high on the glycemic index (over 50). White bread, white potatoes, white pasta, white rice, and other refined grains are rapidly broken down into glucose, which stimulates the release of insulin in your system. This white trash ultimately results in altered blood sugar levels and may lead to weight gain and heart disease.

The following members of the evil empire are the arch nemeses of your time around the table. They're a rough crowd. If these guys are your friends, who needs enemies? I'm being light, but be serious about your healthy lifestyle change. You'll need to go through your cupboards, pantry, and fridge and do some soul searching. What I did the last time was, first, I went through all the food I had in the house noting everything that shouldn't be there, then I wrote up a menu using ALL of it and threw a party for family and friends. I sent home all the leftovers with them. This way I was ready to make a clean break with those bad guys—kind of a farewell party to my old ways! The day after your party, go out and shop till you drop, using your MyTendWell Shopping List, buying only items on the Tremendous 20 list (chap. 4), and you'll be victorious over the evil empire immediately. Try it. Sometimes it takes doing something novel to send a message to both yourself and those around you that you're trying something new and you need their support. So . . . here are the evil empire cast of characters.

White Flour

Giving up white flour feels, for me, like a heroin addict in a methadone clinic. It is always around you, tempting you both out in the open and lurking in the dark alleys. White flour is in many of our favorite foods. Most muffins, pizzas, pancakes, breads, bagels, pastries, and crackers have white flour as their major ingredient. But white is also hiding for a sneak attack. It adds richness and thickness to soups, stews, gravies, and sauces. It binds bisques and gives pasta its voluptuous body. It hasn't always been this way. Widespread use of white flour is an invention of the modern times. Our forefathers used mostly whole grains for their cooking. The problem with refined flour is that it's a simple carbohydrate that almost instantly turns to sugar in the digestive process and then is stored as fat unless we

White flour is what is left over after the processing of wheat has stripped the grain off the bran and germ leaving just the endosperm. Unfortunately, the bran and germ are the most nutrient dense parts of wheat. Further, much of today's wheat (as well as corn, soybean, and sugar cane) crops are sprayed with Roundup®, a herbicide containing glyphosate, which may be the real culprit of celiac disease, and more common gluten intolerance.

Research suggests that glyphosate is a major cause of obesity, autism, Alzheimer's, Parkinson's, infertility, kidney failure, depression, and cancer. Glyphosate is an antimicrobial and therefore wreaks havoc on digestive tracks human and nonhuman, killing off those healthy microbes or gut bacteria. In fact, to read the research on glyphosate makes me want to grow and hoe for the rest of my life and eat nothing but what I grow and preserve.

are not extremely active. Read your labels and avoid foods, even foods that say "whole wheat," if enriched flour is first on the list of ingredients.

White Sugar

In the relative history of humankind, white sugar, as we know it, was developed in the past 30 seconds. This shows that we've been living without it for millions of years and really don't need it. But we love it. We are addicted to it. The problem with sugar is much like that of flour. It raises our blood glucose levels and gives us a high. Usually the rush leaves us crashing and burning soon after and in need of another fix. What can we do to satisfy the sweet tooth? Turn to fresh seasonal fruit, dried fruits, fruit purees, sugar-free fruit sorbets, agave nectar, sweet spices, vanilla beans, and honey (which is used

> **Sinful Sugar:** When discussing food and eating behaviors, I typically tell my clients that the road to hell is paved with sugar. It's the ultimate smack! And we are junkies for junk food. You know the challenge of cutting out those sugary snacks and sweets. Sugar is everywhere and you are tempted at every turn. But fight that temptation. Sugar is not good for us. It provides only calories and no nutrients. And although it is a challenge, keep sugar to a minimum.
>
> **Another important note:** Sugar is also treated with glyphosate. Sugar-industry workers are exposed to glyphosate and have a high incidence of kidney failure.

by our bodies much like sugar but at least has other beneficial qualities and great flavor). The idea is to get some fiber and other benefits from the sweet foods we eat and to stay away from "empty" calories that send fat to waistlines, and other places. If you try to use these healthy sweets 90 percent of the time, you will feel better about that occasional chocolate soufflé when you have a night on the town. Chocoholic? Try darker and somewhat bitter varieties. You'll find you can be satisfied with the more sophisticated flavor and less of it.

White Rice

Nothing goes with Chinese takeout like that sticky white rice that comes with it. I always order both brown and white rice but the white rice is always the first to go. Brown rice just doesn't take to the sauce the same way. I personally love brown rice, but it did take me a while to grow accustomed to it. I love using the leftovers for making a salad or stir-fries the next day. Our digestive system processes white rice the same way as white flour, turning it directly into sugar, which can be stored as fat. Don't make the

mistake of thinking that those crispy rice cakes are any better. Long the drug of choice for health food junkies, these cakes raise your glycemic index just like sugar and flour do.

> **Quick Tip:** To remove the maximum amount of toxins, rinse rice well before cooking and cook it in plenty of water. Chef D recommends a 6:1 ratio of water to rice. Drain excess water, season to taste and enjoy!

> **Rice** is a potential source of arsenic. Arsenic is a naturally occurring metal found in the soil and water. Rice, grown in paddies in which the rice is submerged in water, absorbs the arsenic. White basmati rice (California, India, and Pakistan) has been found to have about half the arsenic. Brown basmati rice (California, India, and Pakistan) has about a third less.

Excessive Alcohol (White Lightning)

Most chefs love to drink. It is often the nature of the business. We work hard and we play hard. We create wonderful experiences and memories for others, pampering and spoiling our guests nightly without taking the time to even treat

> **How you metabolize alcohol**
> depends on gender, race, physical size and condition, as well as whether food is in the stomach or other medication present. Additionally, the production of alcohol dehydrogenase, an enzyme used in alcohol metabolism, contributes to breaking down alcohol. Importantly, women do not metabolize alcohol like men do in part because of the lower activity of alcohol dehydrogenase in the stomach lining.

ourselves to a sit-down meal. After midnight, when the guests have all been served dessert, we often have our only meal of the day (usually containing white flour, white rice, sugar, and plenty of salt), and it is often accompanied by several glasses of a favorite wine or beer. We then head home, shower, and hit the hay . . . unless there is some leftover ice cream in the freezer. Alcohol reacts like the other sugars on this list. It also inhibits our ability to resist temptations.

Excessive Sodium

Salt is necessary for life. You can read all about it in a fabulous book by Mark Kurlansky titled *SALT*. The problem is excess. Again, read labels and remember what I say to cooking staff: "You can always add a bit more at the table, but once it is in there you can't take it out." If you are a salt-aholic, try weaning yourself by not seasoning while you are cooking. Rather, just finish with a pinch of those big crunchy crystals of high-quality sea salt. These give you that salt "fix" without overdoing it.

> **Sodium** intake has long been associated with hypertension and water retention. There is some research investigating the use of low-sodium diets to control asthma. Replace salting your food by spicing it up with herbs and spices, many of which have health benefits of their own. Or use Chef D's trick. Sprinkle coarse salts, like Brittany, at the end of cooking or just before serving individual dishes.

Hidden Fats

Did you know that French fries are really Belgian, and the best French fries are traditionally cooked in horse fat? Enough said? These rendered fats, which usually congeal into a solid white block at room temperature, are really tasty, until you

think about it. They are mostly calories without the benefits of the protein you get when eating the animal muscle from which the fats are extracted. Humans have used these fats forever, and when every calorie was precious to conserve and consume, the more the better. But today, with our more sedentary lifestyles, we can't continue to eat the way our more physically active (think up at dawn and down at dusk with only farm work in between) forefathers did. Fat is good. We need fat to live and to absorb maximum nutritional benefits from our foods. If you are using fat, use real fat and enjoy it. The fats I'm speaking of are the hidden fats in many of the processed foods we eat without even recognizing it.

> **Fats** are essential for the regulation of fat-soluble vitamins A, D, E, and K. Fat is important in the protection of organs. Fat is also higher in calories per gram. Where carbohydrates and protein provide four calories per gram, fat provides more than twice that at nine calories per gram. This is important in nutrition planning to determine the percentage of calories per nutrient: for example, 60 percent carbohydrates, 25 percent protein, and 15 percent fat.

Refined White Starches

Potato flour, cornstarch, and white rice flour are used in cooking all over the world much the same way we use wheat flour. They are made into rice paper and wonton wrappers and used for thickening stir-fries, sauces, soups, and stews. These are hidden starches that we don't usually know we are eating when we order dishes in restaurants and from delivery menus. Again, starches are good, but I am talking about the empty calories in most baked goods in the supermarket and the packaged food available in this country's "food deserts." It seems that the wealthier we are, the more able we are to eat like cavemen. We can find and afford unrefined whole foods like artisanal (expensive) whole-grain pastas, sprouted-grain breads, rediscovered ancient foods like freekeh and farro, and imported whole-grain crisps and crackers.

> Simple **carbohydrates** are what we need to limit. Simple carbs or sugars and starches are simply combined molecules that are quick to metabolize and thus do not provide sustainable energy. Work to replace simple carbs with complex carbs found in whole grains. There are lots of grains. Try some different varieties that are organic and non-GMO. These foods add more flavor per chew—so slow down the process and enjoy the added textures and nutrients.

Fatty Dairy Products

Dairy is not a dirty word, but we need to stick mostly to the lower-fat varieties. Lower-fat and no-fat varieties of yogurts, milk, sour cream, and cheeses are great for everyday dining. Nonfat ricotta cheese can be used for stuffings, dips, and desserts. Try soy and almond cheeses as well as tofu sour cream and cream cheese. When it comes to butter, I choose the real thing, using it when olive oil can't be substituted. Save that triple cream brie for a special occasion when you have enough people around so everyone gets just one bite and none is left tempting you in the cheese drawer. Yes, I have a cheese drawer.

> **Fats in dairy products** can be up to 50 percent of the calories provided, such as in whole milk. This amount of fat can be reduced by using low-fat dairy products.

Processed Foods

These are one of the biggest problems in kitchens today. I believe that these foods, especially the ones labeled fat-free or sugar-free, not only taste terrible but allow you to feel that you have a safe binge food you can pig out on. If you really want a treat you should go for the best and have the real thing. Make sure you become a label reader. I spent 15 minutes reading peanut butter labels the other day to find one that didn't have sugar as the second ingredient. Processed foods usually have a lot of chemical preservatives as well. A simple rule that I follow from Michael Pollen is if you can't pronounce it and your gramma wouldn't have known what it is, don't buy it. Just remember that the only way you can lose weight and maintain your loss is with a balance of healthy eating and proper daily movement. There is no magic way to get healthy and if something sounds too good to be true, it probably isn't true.

> **Processed foods** are high in calories and low in nutrients. The grains are stripped of their nutrients and left with the simple starch. Generally cheap and well marketed, these foods have become the staples in our diets. A good strategy for avoiding these foods is to shop the perimeter of the grocery. Typically processed foods are in the center aisles, so fill your cart with the items found in the outskirts or perimeter—like fresh produce.

Fried Crispy Snacks

These can be a downfall—potato chips, nachos, fried plantains, egg rolls, tempuras, and, of course, French fries. Most of these snacks are built around refined starches that you have already learned are our archenemies. Now, drop them in a hot vat of fat. Do you really think that will make them any healthier? An old nemesis was the cocktail hour. I love a good scotch or two, but one has to set priorities. Alcoholic drinks break down the control system and one ends up eating many of these greasy snacks—and that's all before sitting down to dinner. It's so much better to start off with some hummus and crudités served with an herbal iced tea. Have one glass of red wine with your meal and you're good to go!

> **Fried foods, fast foods,** and many processed foods are produced and prepared with hydrogenated and trans fats. These are fats that have been modified by the process of adding hydrogen to unsaturated fats in order to change the properties of these fats to be more solid and spreadable.

Hydrogenated and Trans Fats

These are the nasty fats that clog the digestive system with greasy plaque blockages. Hydrogen is added to make liquid oils solid. They are used to make things tender or crispy and are meant to last on store shelves for months and months. They are not natural in our diets or even in nature. Get away from them! Don't walk, *run*! If you are going to have a chocolate chip cookie have a real chocolate chip cookie. These trans fats should be avoided at all costs.

> These food items are always found in the center of the store . . . and the end caps of the isles, at the checkout, and so on and so on. What restaurant doesn't offer fries as a side? **Convenient foods** are a downfall for most of us. Snack foods often have us thinking we aren't eating too much, but we are really just packing in empty calories. Chef D and Dr. K promote in their MyTendWell Lifestyle Plan five small meals per day.

Preservatives and Pesticides

Avoid processed foods containing chemical preservatives. If what you read on the label isn't something that can be grown or raised, you should probably leave it on the supermarket shelf. Pesticides are the chemicals used to treat plants that are under siege by pests. Sounds tasty! Many manmade pesticides are systemic and are absorbed by food sources and afterward by us. You can't wash them off. Choose to go organic whenever possible. Organic may be somewhat more expensive but well worth a few cents more if you can possibly afford it. If organic produce isn't available at your market ask the manager about it. The more we assert a desire for this type of product the more competition there will be, often driving prices down. Get off your chemical dependency!

> The control of weeds and pests in the growing of food products, such as wheat and corn, with the use of **chemical herbicides and pesticides** has become standard operating procedure in farming. These chemicals, often synthetic estrogens, are dangerous to health and may be mediators in the development of cancers. Therefore, limit foods that may be produced this way. Buy and eat organic when available. Better yet, try to buy local food products grown by local farmers . . . or grow your own. Then you definitely know what you are eating.

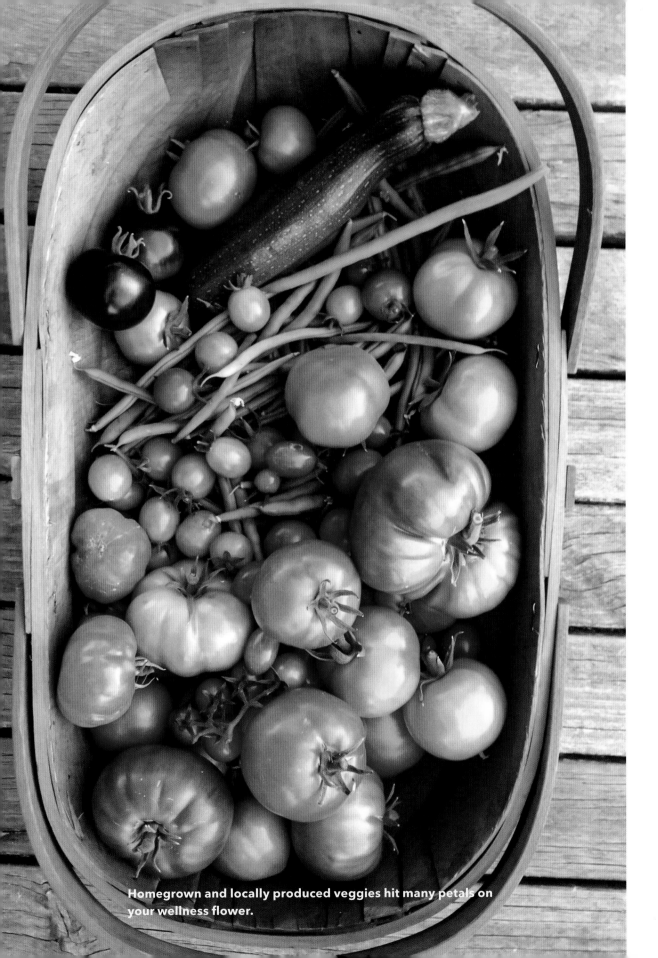

Homegrown and locally produced veggies hit many petals on your wellness flower.

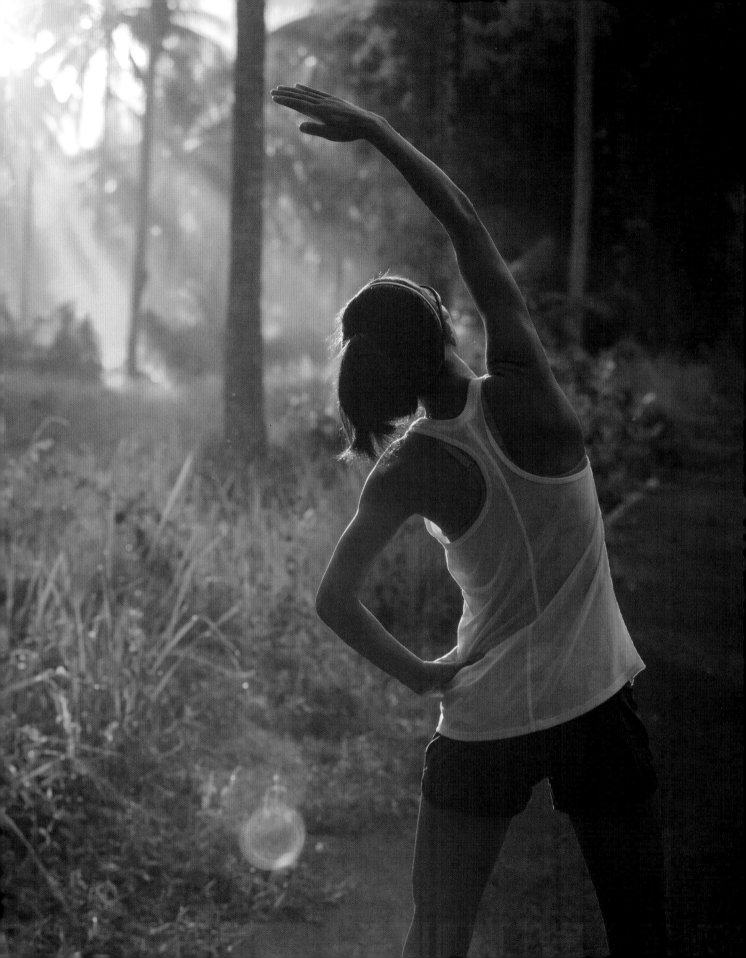

3

Cultivating a New You

FINDING BALANCE IN THIS SHAKY NEW WORLD

If one is not living by the old adages "Everything in moderation" and "You are what you eat," then understanding the art of balance may be difficult to achieve. But, in reality, those two old sayings ring as true as they always have. In the Midwestern grain belt, our traditional family gatherings and holidays are full of dishes that were developed for fuel. Farmers and farmhands were fed huge amounts of starchy, carbo-filled foods, perfect for providing them the energy to do hard work by hand in the fields. When the family got together, there were big bowls of chicken and dumplings, grits with cheese, biscuits with sausage gravy, fried chicken, icebox cakes, pies, and cobblers, all of which are delicious but not for daily consumption in today's office cubical work world. In the past there was a balance of food to fuel bodies engaged in hard physical labor on the farm. Now that most of the work done on farms is done by machine, even farmers need to think about food balance in their lives, saving the everyday dishes of the past for special occasions!

In big cities like New York, Chicago, and L.A. things are even more difficult and hectic. Finding balance and achieving satisfaction from this middle of the highway swinging pendulum is practically impossible. After a day of stressful work in a big city, saying, "I'll only have one bite

or one beer," or one of anything, for that matter, is tough. Finding balance is not just about having one of anything or eliminating a food that you enjoy completely from your life. It's about understanding the relationship between what you put in your mouth and balancing that fuel, in a healthy lifestyle, with movement. It is essential to remember what you've eaten earlier in the day and the day before, and then to structure upcoming meals and healthy movement to achieve balance. It is OK to play, but you have to remember to pay. Everything has a cost.

We've all heard our parents or grandparents ranting, "When I was your age we didn't have so much on the table, so you better eat everything." Or, "We didn't have shoes to walk to school in, so appreciate the advantages you have now." In actuality, they may have had the advantage because there was less processed food, less day-to-day stress, and, for most, a more structured family life. Today's children grow up putting a package of unnatural food in the microwave and calling it dinner. Kids, not to mention adults, skip breakfast or eat "cereal and milk bars"; eat pizza, burgers and fries, frozen processed snacks, and hotdogs. They drink milk pumped with hormones and antibiotics; but mostly they drink high fructose corn syrup sweetened fizzy water with "artificial flavorings." Is this really getting the most out of life? It's difficult to think about achieving balance when the pendulum has swung so far away from nature and seems to be

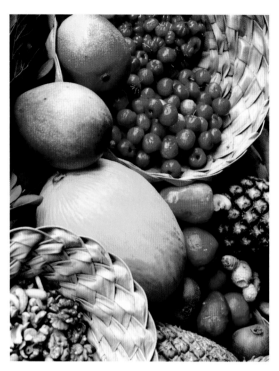

Brazilian cornucopia: mangoes, acerola, cashews with cashew apple, pineapple, ginger, kiwi, walnuts, and melon.

stuck on the side of processed convenience. To really create balance, we need to think about moving our bodies, eating organic foods, cooking at home, and stress relief, and we need to rethink our goals. As a country we waste and throw away more food than any other in the world. This is reprehensible. We need to figure out a way to share our food, and our strength, both as families and as humans, and not continue to overbuy, overspend, overeat, and waste our food.

Most kids don't learn how to cook anymore; their mothers and dads don't cook! When I teach cooking to kids, many can't tell the difference between arugula and zucchini; to them they are just vegetables. Sixty-seven percent of the American diet consists of potatoes (instant, fried, potato chips, "tots," and fresh), iceberg lettuce, tomatoes (mostly canned), carrots, and onions. Whatever happened to standard stuff like broccoli, Brussels sprouts, watercress, or even asparagus? As culinary ambassadors, chefs have tried to expose the public to new exotic and old heirloom varieties of fruits and vegetables for years. Some have caught on and have become standard items in grocery stores in big cities, but small town America is often still a wasteland unless you grow things yourself. I read a quote in the *New York Times* stating the average American ate 7.7 pounds of cheese in the 1950s and now consumes 30 pounds annually. Most of this is not very interesting stuff, it's industrially produced processed cheese—"food" that is used on tacos, pizza, nachos, fast-food hamburgers, and frozen foods, and we wonder why our butts are getting big. Being a citizen of the most obese nation in the world isn't something I'm proud of, but, as a chef, I still create plenty of artery-clogging food because I need to put butts in seats. I must give guests what they want, in portions they feel are giving them good value. Sometimes I'd love to cook better, higher quality, ingredients in reasonable portions, but, an undereducated public would not find the value in that and would go elsewhere. Chefs and restaurant goers need to develop a general understanding of balancing healthy cooking and eating and then teach this to the next generation. Balance is just a heartbeat or . . . a heart attack away.

Nature has provided us with a veritable cornucopia of fruits, vegetables, fish, fowl, nuts, seeds, and berries and much more. There are so many wonderful and surprising natural things that it is hard to believe a heaven could be better. Where are these foods in the average American diet? Usually, even if available, not even put in the shopping cart. We are taught by advertisers what to eat, not by farmers and nutritionists. We reach for the quickest thing to shove into our face, not the healthiest. We let our kids tell us what to buy, not teach them how to cook and eat. It is time for a change, folks.

Moderation is knowing that when you have a hankering for something that wouldn't necessarily be healthy, like a burger and fries for example, and you have to have it, buy the best quality you can afford, take your time to enjoy it to the fullest, then follow your splurge with a commitment to spend extra time moving. Don't waste any time getting back on the healthy eating bandwagon. A balanced diet is made up of fresh vegetables in a rainbow of colors, fruits, fish, lean meats, low-fat dairy products, nuts and seeds, and a good glass of wine or quality beer. To achieve balance is to understand moderation. To understand moderation you have to educate yourself and take advantage of all the wonderful ingredients that are out there. Consume a wide variety in appropriate amounts. Tasting the first Macoun apple or the first soft-shell crab of the season is a splendid experience that one can look forward to with pleasurable anticipation. You don't need to eat foods that are out of season from halfway around the world. Enjoy the fresh local bounty out of your backdoor or local farmers' market. How can today's children or yesterday's adults learn about the rainbow of foods available if we, as chefs, parents, friends, and lovers, don't find this knowledge important enough to share? When people are educated about food and health, finding balance is not such a difficult task. Shopping and cooking are tasks, but they don't have to be chores. Find joy in cooking and eating and share that with others. We are all potential guides in this new adventure of creating a healthy balanced life for ourselves and the ones we care about. Food is medicine; movement is life.

DETOXING AND CREATING A HARMLESS HOME

Just as moderation is key to keeping caloric intake in check, and can help with getting a balance of nutrients from a variety of healthful foods, moderation is also helpful in reducing exposure to environmental contaminants. Foods, beauty products, house furnishings, and various other household products contain a variety of toxins. Exposure to these toxins leads to our bodies storing up a brew of harmful chemicals

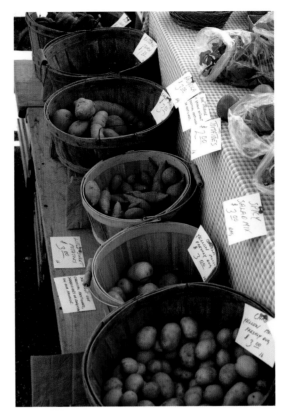

Fall market with potatoes.

and heavy metals. And amassing this brew of toxins is detrimental not just to our own health but especially to the health of the little ones we are bringing up in our world. Thus, as the best defense is a good offense, have a plan of attack—be proactive. Reduce your exposure to these environmental pollutants by controlling what you eat and what you bring into your home. Try growing what you can and knowing what went into the growing process of your food, buy organic, and buy fewer plastic-packaged products.

As discussed in chapter 2, repeated herbicide and pesticide applications on farm fields, lawns, and golf courses contribute to the buildup of toxins in produce, soil, and water; and animal production processes provide yet another source of contamination. Thus, just as toxins build up in our environment and food sources, toxins, similarly, build up in our bodies from these repeated and various sources of exposures. Consequently,

> # We do not inherit the earth from our ancestors, we borrow it from our children.
> —Native American Proverb

for the next generations, the accumulation of toxins will be a bigger concern because there are more toxins in today's environment than in the past. The importance of detoxifying may become more necessary for younger generations. However, researchers have some catching up to do investigating the efficacy of detox diets and drinks, as data is limited.

Age-old detoxification methods from both Native Americans and the Far Easterners are becoming more commonly used to help eliminate the toxicity in our bodies. These include drinks such as dark fruit smoothies, beverages made with turmeric and ginger, kombucha, kvass, and traditional and herbal teas made from green leaves and herbs. Weeds, like dandelions, thistles, and others, are purported to be possible powerhouses of detox and can also be made into teas and infusions. But is detoxing a valid practice? Doesn't our body do this on its own? Yes, in fact it does. The liver, kidneys, gastrointestinal system, lungs, and skin all aid in the elimination of toxins from our body via urine, feces, and sweat. In fact, this is a primary job of these organs to remove foreign substances. The human body is generally quite good at maintaining a balance. This is known as homeostasis.

However, there is concern that the exceedingly high amount of toxins we are exposed to is more than our systems can handle. Just as our brain has a fixed capacity for information processing, our body has only so much energy for its numerous physiological processes. How we allocate this energy to accomplish these physiological processes is important. Consider when you are dealing with a cold or flu. Your body will need a little more energy to fight the bug that is attacking your body. This energy will most likely be borrowed from another need.

Homeostasis: French physiologist Claud Bernard (1813–1878) referred to the human body's amazing ability to maintain a constant internal environment regardless of the external environment as *milieu intérieur*. Later, American physiologist Walter Cannon (1871–1945) called this ability *homeostasis*. He then put forward that the goal of all of the body's physiological regulations was the "maintenance of internal constancy." A good example of this is body temperature. Normal (i.e., the mean or average, within the population) body temperature is 98.6 (yes, there is variance. I indicated normal is the mean . . . everything always goes back to the mean). Thus, when we go to the doctor, our temperature is taken and 98.6 is the baseline from which to tell if we are running a fever.

Regulation of body temperature is one of the many systems and processes our bodies maintain; others are, for instance, menstruation, cardiac rhythm, breathing, hormonal balance, and gut bacteria. Yes, good gut bacteria help the intestines break down foods. Our bodies host bacteria that produce enzymes to break down foods during digestion. Research has demonstrated that glyphosate (a chemical in Roundup) interferes with the digestion of foods by disrupting the functioning of cytochrome P450 enzymes.

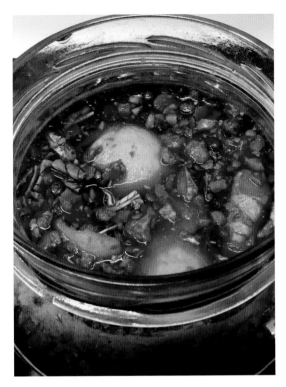

Beet, orange, and kimchi kvass with allspice.

This is the same philosophy with detoxing in that detoxing methods may be beneficial in assisting our body with what is a natural process. More simply put, if your body is "toxic," your systems mentioned above will need to work to clean it up. If we are able to utilize detoxing methods, such as kvass, then this assistance could decrease the work of our body's natural detoxing processes.

But does drinking a tea or eating herbs provide assistance with detoxing? Currently there is no research supporting the use of commercial detox treatments. There is some evidence that the nutritional properties of some foods are beneficial. For instance, acids found in fruits, such as citric acid (citrus fruits), succinic acid (apples and blueberries), as well as citrus pectin (fruit peels) and chlorella (green algae) assist in chelating toxic metals from our bodies. We must stop looking at the natural environment as an opponent to defeat and instead thank Mother Nature for her gifts.

Quick Tips for Eating Organic

Lemons: We typically put lemon slices or wedges in drinks or on food. If your lemons have been sprayed with a pesticide or herbicide, likely those are still in the rind. Buy organic lemons so when you are flavoring your iced tea, you are just getting flavor, not a little chemical tea bag.

Lettuces, spinaches, kale: We want that fresh salad all year long, so try growing your own. Get an oblong-shaped planter, one that will sit in front of or in the sill of a window that gets some good sun exposure, plant some of your favorite salad mixes, and watch them grow. You can put a little plastic over the planter to create a greenhouse effect to get your veggies started. Then you know what is in your produce.

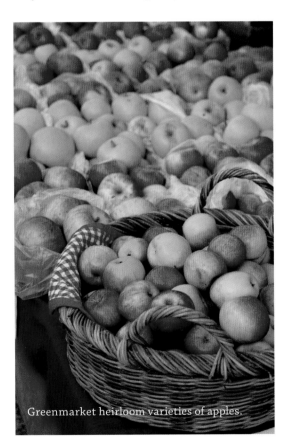

Greenmarket heirloom varieties of apples.

THE BEST AND THE WORST OF SUPERMARKET PRODUCE

Pick organic versions from the first list and, if on a budget, nonorganic varieties from the second. Soft-skinned fruits and vegetables on list #1 have the hardest time with pests, so they are usually the ones we put the most poisons on. Notice that many of the foods in list #2 have thick, inedible skins surrounding and protecting the fruit or vegetable. These are thought to be the ones you can choose nonorganic versions of.

BUY ORGANIC

- apples
- bell peppers
- celery
- cherries
- grapes—86 percent of imported grapes (i.e., Chile) sampled were found to contain pesticides
- nectarines
- peaches
- pears
- potatoes
- red raspberries
- spinach
- strawberries
- tomatoes

CONVENTIONAL OKAY

- asparagus
- avocados
- bananas
- broccoli
- cauliflower
- corn
- kiwi
- mangoes
- onions
- papaya
- pineapples
- sweet peas (shelled)

TEAS

Teas are broken down into two variet-teas . . . (tea joke).

True teas are made from the tea plant, which naturally contains caffeine. These come in many varieties from different growing regions and processing techniques. All black and green teas are true teas. These may also be flavored with various herbs, spices, and flavorings.

Herbal teas are made with no true tea and are almost exclusively caffeine free. Herbs teas have been used as folk medicine around the world for generations. Modern medicine is finally catching up with our ancestors and accepting the value of many of the plant potions.

The antioxidants in these teas are of great benefit to health, from the relaxation properties of lavender and chamomile to the gastric intestinal motility stimulator of senna tea.

Chef D's childhood lake home is a testament to gardening perseverance. Chef D's mother, Mary Lu, has created a landscape that is aesthetically amazing and palatable. Some of the rare treats are the elder bushes. Chef D and Dr. K harvest the flowers and the berries for teas. Elder flower and berry tea aid respiratory function.

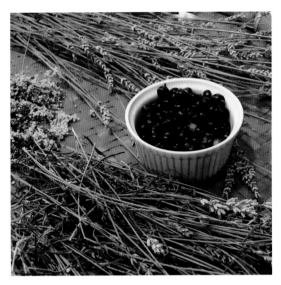

Chef D and Dr. K's crop for herb and berry tea.

MyTendWell CHALLENGE

Grow and Dry
Your Own Herbs

Start simple. Oregano, parsley, and basil are easy to grow in a small garden or patio planter. Cut, tie into small bundles, and hang upside down by the kitchen sink or a window to dry. Once dry, store in a glass container with a lid in a dark, cool place.

PLAY PADS, MATS, AND BLANKETS FOR THE INFANTS IN YOUR LIFE

Little ones need to have some room to roam—this encourages movement. Put a little tyke on the floor and before you know it, they are rolling over, creeping, and crawling. They try and try and try to pick things up, to get to their toys—all the good stuff that gives them experiences that enhance learning and development. But what's on the floor? More than you probably prefer to know and more than what the little one needs to be exposed to. Get a play pad, mat, or blanket that you can pack and go so your precious little one is best protected. Chemical residue from lawn applications, dirt and disease from the sidewalks, animal waste from the dog run or horse barn, and other contaminants we don't like to think about are all tracked in to the infant's environment. We also add cleaning products, dust, dander, fragrances, and other toxins to our homes that we might not consider. So, when young children are in your home, put a barrier between their bums and your floor.

SUNSCREEN

Outdoor activities are a favorite of mine—all year long. I play in the snow and dig in the dirt—all under a big, bright sun. I'm also fair-skinned, and Chef D is a darling ginger, so protecting our skin is important. I lather up all year with a good sunscreen and get skin cancer screens. Check with your doctor or hospital; there may be free skin cancer screenings available to you. When making a sunscreen selection, pick one with zinc oxide and sun protection factor (SPF) of at least 15, preferably 30. And don't forget the shades. Sun protection for your eyes is especially important in preventing cataracts. Tomatoes contain lycopene, which is a natural sunscreen, so make sure you eat plenty.

HOME MIXTURES, REMEDIES, AND CONCOCTIONS

VINEGAR—A GREAT ALL-PURPOSE ITEM

Fly Spray

Dr. K uses this on her horses: Mix equal parts of apple cider vinegar, pine cleaner, and a few drops of dish soap. Keep in a labeled spray bottle.

Air Freshener

Mix ¼ cup white vinegar, ¾ cup water, and 5–10 drops of your favorite essential oil—lavender, cinnamon, lemongrass (very nice)—whatever suits you. Keep in a labeled spray bottle.

Odor Reducer

Mix equal parts white vinegar and water; spray on fabrics, on rugs and carpets (home and car), and in refrigerators and coolers.

Drain Cleaner

Sprinkle baking soda at the drain opening, and pour white vinegar over baking soda. Let mixture work down the drain. Rinse with hot water and repeat if necessary. (This also helps with spots in clothes, fabrics, and carpets.)

Weed Spray

In a large spray bottle, mix 1 quart white vinegar, 1–2 teaspoons of biodegradable liquid dish soap, and 4–5 teaspoons of clove oil. Store in a spray bottle for up to one year.

SKIN ABRASIONS, BURNS AND WOUNDS

Bee Sting Paste

Running barefoot was commonplace growing up in Ogilville, Indiana, for Chef D and Dr. K, and stepping on honey bees was just a part of summer. Our home remedy was a paste of baking soda and water. As beekeepers, Chef D and Dr. K still get stung. They put a spin on the old home remedy by adding a bit of essential oil. Chef D likes lavender; Dr. K prefers it with lemongrass.

Mix 1 teaspoon of baking soda, 2 drops of essential oil and a few drops of distilled water to form a paste. Apply to sting and leave on. Paste will dry and flake off. Reapply if needed. (Makes enough for one application.)

Look for organic and biofriendly products at your local supermarket; they usually have them all in the same area. Also go online and do a quick search for any type of household product you are looking for. They will usually be easy to make (use products you already have on hand), and be much less expensive than the name brands you have been using.

Aloe Vera

Those houseplants aren't just for decoration. They oxygenate your home, add color, and give you useful products. Aloe vera is great in mixtures or all alone. Keep one or two plants in your care all year long.

Soothe a Burn

Grow an aloe vera plant or two and you'll have a bit of medicinal gel for burns. Cut off a leaf, and squeeze gel onto burn. Repeat as necessary.

Skin Spritz

Mix ½ cup aloe vera juice, ½ teaspoon of essential oil (lavender, tea tree, peppermint, lemongrass), and 1 tablespoon of apple cider vinegar. Mix well and keep refrigerated in spray bottle. This works well on sunburns, too.

Massage Gel

Mix 1–2 ounces of aloe vera gel and 6–10 drops of your favorite essential oil in a small jar, cover and shake to mix. Store in a cool place for up to one year.

Cleansing Hand Gel

In small, tight-sealing jar, mix 1–2 ounces of aloe vera gel with 8–10 drops of tea tree oil. Store for up to one year.

Honey

Wound Care

Not only is honey sweet to taste and healthful to eat; it is also a bacteria-fighting aid and can be applied straight from the jar to cuts and scrapes to soothe and heal them.

MOISTURIZERS, CLEANSERS AND SCRUBS

Nail and Cuticle Scrub

Mix 1 tablespoon of honey, 1 tablespoon of sea salt, 1 tablespoon of essential oil (tea tree, almond, peppermint, lavender), and 1 tablespoon of witch hazel extract. Massage into each nail and cuticle, then rinse with warm water. Moisturize with hand and foot cream after.

Hand and Foot Cream

Chef D and Dr. K are always getting down and dirty . . . in the garden, in the kitchen, and with the bee hives. Their hands and feet take a beating. So, with the beeswax they get from their hives, they refresh dry, tired skin with an easy to make cream.

Melt ½ cup of cocoa butter and ½ cup of beeswax in a double boiler. Add 1 tablespoon of your favorite essential oil (lavender, tea tree, lemongrass), then add a few drops of vitamin E oil (squeeze 3–4 capsules or buy in liquid form).

Pour and store mixture in a glass jar. (Dr. K likes to use shallow, wide-mouth jelly jars.) Let cool before sealing with lid. These make great gifts, and it's fun to decorate jars with labels and lid covers.

Facial Cleanser

Pour a little extra-virgin olive oil onto fingertips; massage and clean face.

Facial Toner

Pour ¼ cup (2 oz.) of witch hazel in a sealable jar. Add rosemary essential oil (lavender, chamomile). After cleansing face, apply with cotton ball. Rosemary helps relax and calm.

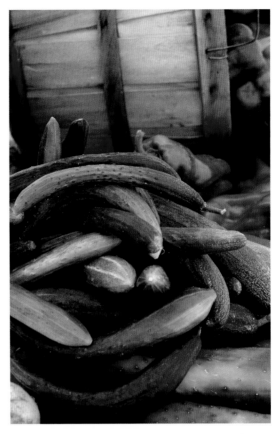

Cool as a cucumber. These are great for refreshing facial masks.

Shop the antiques and uniques stores and look for a nifty apothecary jar with a tight-fitting lid to store your toner and oils in.

FACIAL MASKS

Avocado Mask

Mash ½ of an avocado with ¼ cup of honey, apply to skin, and leave on for 10 minutes. Rinse with cool water.

Cucumber Mask

Cut 4 disks from a homegrown cucumber, grate the rest. Lightly squeeze grated cucumber, mix in fresh mint, lemon verbena, lavender, and 2 tablespoons of thick yogurt. Place disks over relaxed eyes, and spread mixture over skin. Leave on while you relax for 30 minutes.

MOISTURIZER FOR HAIR AND SKIN

Mix coconut or extra-virgin olive oil and your favorite essential oil (rosemary, lavender, or lemon verbena) in a tight-sealing jar. Store for up to three months.

For dry skin: rub onto skin after warm bath

For split ends: rub into hair and leave on overnight. Wash out in morning. This is better than the old "hot-oil" treatments Mom used to do.

MOISTURIZING SHAMPOO

In one of your new "old" (tightly sealing) jars that you found at the antiques store, mix ½ cup liquid castile soap, ¼ cup glycerin, and ¼ cup of coconut oil. Add your favorite essential oil (tea tree, sweet almond, peppermint). Shake to mix. Store up to three months.

TOOTHPASTE

Mix baking soda and a bit of hydrogen peroxide, dip toothbrush into mixture, brush, and rinse.

BREATH FRESHENER

Bring 2 cups of water with dried leaves of mint (peppermint, spearmint), rosemary, and fennel seeds to a boil. Let cool and keep in refrigerator for about a week. Swish for fresh breath.

BREATH FRESHENING TOOTHPICKS

Fill the bottom of a shot glass with tea tree oil (*Melaleuca alternifolia*), place wood toothpicks in the shot glass and let soak up the tea tree oil. Store toothpicks in small glass jar. Tea tree oil is antiseptic, antibacterial, antifungal, and antiviral and is therefore great at fighting germs and infections.

DEODORANT

Combine ½ cup of cornstarch and ½ cup of baking soda, add 2–3 drops of tea tree oil, mix well and store in a glass jar with a tight-sealing lid. Use a powder puff to apply under arms.

PETS

Pets are great friends and companions; they lift your spirits and make your life better. Many hospitals and rehab centers are using pet therapy to help patients recover more quickly. In fact, Dr. K's dog, Louie, was her little companion during chemotherapy. He'd sleep at her feet when she was "laid-up" in bed.

Having a pet can also be like having a workout partner. A dog can give you a reason to get out of bed in the morning. All you have to do is take the next step: put a leash on your dog and take it for a walk. Knowing that there is another living thing waiting for you to give it food, water, attention, exercise, and companionship can get you through those darker days.

Chef D's twin tuxedo cats, Connor and Cooper, have often made a lonely home into a three-ring circus with their hijinks and late-night yowling.

Even a fish tank, ant farm, snake, lizard, or bird can give someone fighting a bout of loneliness a sense of community.

HOBBY "PETS"

Dr. K and Chef D both are beekeepers, and although it may not be a daily chore 365 days a year, the bees do need attention. They are also a break from your normal routine and get you thinking about nature and the outdoors, which can be a stress reliever. Yes, the bees can be tricky, but they teach you about moving slowly and thoughtfully and with purpose. There is almost a Zen practice to the task. But if you don't have the space or desire for the hobby, you might think about other hobbies that include animals. Horseback riding, a chicken or pigeon coop, a butterfly or bee garden, or even a worm farm are all ways to bring the natural world into your life.

Even if you live in a metropolitan area, you can still feed pigeons or go to a petting zoo. Chef D loves to set out birdbaths and feeders for his wild winged friends and watch and listen to the cacophony. Taking a week of vacation "birding" or just a Saturday afternoon nature hike can transform your mental health.

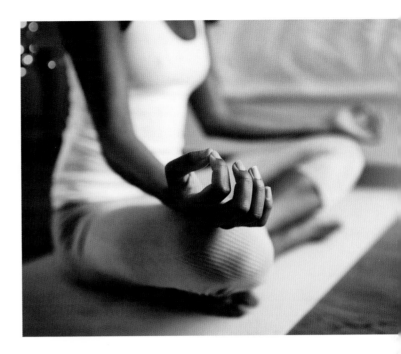

AROMATHERAPY

An alternative form of therapy for stress reduction, relaxation, and sleep improvement, aromatherapy is popular in massage and reflexology and is also used in cancer therapy. It is purported to produce relaxation via the use of essential oils of plants either through skin application or through the olfactory system from infusers. Evidence is sketchy as to the efficacy of aromatherapy, although there are some findings demonstrating reduction in saliva cortisol (remember that stress glucocorticoid?).

Try a bath with some nice aromatherapy; give it a go and see if you notice a difference (more so than a bath without aromatherapy, that is—we need to have rigor in our methodology!).

When someone is sick, make them chicken soup! Just the aroma will make them feel cared for. Also try:

- Try burning dried bay laurel leaves.
- Rosemary is thought to help with memory. Make a tea with honey and lemon and sip slowly while inhaling the aroma through your nose.

- Put mulling spices like cinnamon, cloves, and orange peel in a pot of boiling water and allow it to simmer. The scent will cover cooking and other household smells.

- Keep your spent lemons on the side during cooking. At the end of the day, after everything is clean and put away, run your in-sink garbage disposal with them in it along with some hot tap water. It makes the kitchen smell great and deodorizes your disposal.

- Burn candles in your bathroom. It covers odors and creates a calming space for that long soak you are going to treat yourself to.

MEDITATION

Just as we need to turn ourselves on, we also need to turn ourselves off. In today's digitally stimulated, sugar-jacked mind, we need to "chillax!" Meditation is a great way to turn off—everything.

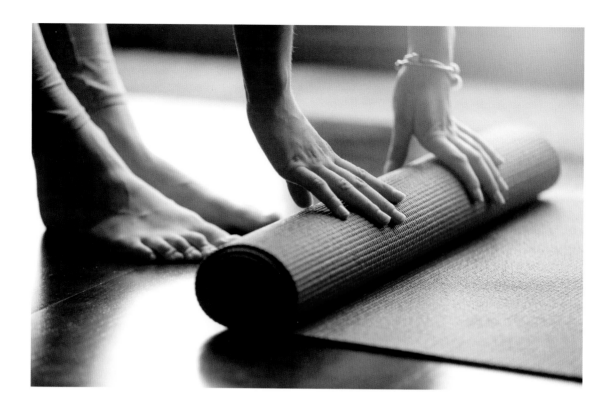

Many of us find going to sleep difficult. We watch television until the wee hours of the night and often end up snacking on sugary, salty, or fatty foods at the end of the day. Sometimes even when we are between the sheets! This is the perfect behavior to replace with meditation.

It is as simple as allowing yourself to lie comfortably on your bed, relaxing all your muscles, clearing your mind, and paying attention to your breathing by inhaling slowly and consistently then exhaling thoroughly. Repeat!

It reads simple, but before you know it you'll be thinking about something at work that day or that date you have tomorrow night. It does take a lot of practice.

Remember all that stuff we told you to turn off earlier? Well, not so fast. . . . There are lots of apps that you can download for meditation training as well as sleep assistance. Download a few for free and try them out. If you find one you like, you can subscribe.

Not into meditation?

You might just try listening to audiobooks with the lights off. We love *Winnie the Pooh*, *Charlotte's Web*, *Grimms' Fairy Tales*, *The Wind in the Willows*, and other nostalgic stories that you already know and don't require your focus. You'll be asleep before you know it.

YOGA, PILATES, AND EASTERN MOVEMENT

Chef D prefers FroGo to yoga . . . but that is a different story.

But honestly, yoga is another way to take yourself out of your head and allow yourself to focus on your body and the environment you are in. Chef's only issue is that it takes time and practice. It might feel uncomfortable or even be a bit difficult in the beginning, but with patience and practice it can be transformative. It stretches your muscles and flexes your joints, creating better blood flow and muscle communication. As you get older, some things become more difficult. Heck, putting on your undies and socks is even a chore. Yoga, Tai Chi, and other fluid movement practices can be important physical and social aspects of your life.

So, try it hot, try it fast—maybe slow—try it with meditation (death pose!). There are lots of options for trying yoga. But remember, yoga is a practice, a discipline that takes years of training. So, if you are new to it, find a good yogi or instructor who has those years of experience and training and will be most likely to teach you, provide feedback, and correct your poses. Videos/DVDs are nice as they are accessible to you at *your* convenience.

Dr. K's tips:

Research your options—ask a friend.

Find an instructor/yogi that has experience and provides feedback about poses and alignment and corrects your form. Any experienced instructor should be able to provide appropriate cues to correct possible mistakes.

Pick something you like and that will engage you.

Schedule your yoga/Pilates workout as you would a doctor's appointment. Just because you have a video/DVD in the house doesn't mean you'll do it. Schedule it!

DOWN (QUIET) TIME

Noise, computers, TVs, traffic! What about some peace and quiet? Studies have demonstrated that time spent quietly can be as effective as meditation and exercise in reducing blood pressure and stress (although exercise provides longer lasting effects in reducing blood pressure).

Known as Distraction Hypothesis, it suggests that exercise, meditation, and quiet time may provide a time-out from things that may be causing stress or anxiety.

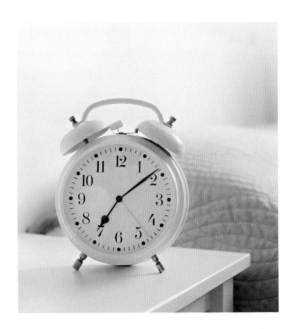

What is important is making the time for quiet. Gardening is a nice quiet time for me. I focus on the plants and the work while listening to wind in the trees and all the native birds singing. I've been learning from Mary Lu (Chef D's mom) the different birdsongs—so I try to identify them as I work in my garden or when I ride my horse—which is great down time.

SLEEP—IT'S WHAT'S FOR HEALTH

In the past 50 years, sleep duration has decreased and, curiously, obesity has increased. Clearly obesity is not a single-factor problem but rather multifactorial, and while most of us easily recognize lack of physical activity and poor diet as contributors to overweight and obesity, seldom do we consider lack of sleep as a factor.

Sleep is related to hormone balance, regulation of glucose (may contribute to diabetes) and body temperature, functioning of the hippocampus, cardiovascular and immune systems, and memory. However, as sleep deprivation is a health risk factor, it is also a modifiable one (i.e., it can be remedied). (See table 3.1 on the recommended amount of sleep for different age groups.)

3.1 Daily Sleep Recommendations

Age group	Recommended hours of sleep per day
Infant: 4–12 months	12–16 hours per 24 hours (including naps)
Toddler: 1–2 years	11–14 hours per 24 hours (including naps)
Preschool: 3–5 years	10–13 hours per 24 hours (including naps)
School age: 6–12 years	9–12 hours per 24 hours
Teen: 13–18 years	8–10 hours per 24 hours
Adult: 18–60 years	7 or more hours per night

Source: Center for Disease Control

Here are a few sleep tips from Dr. K:

Turn off the tech—don't go to bed with the TV on. Some evidence suggests that a backlit screen interrupts sleep. So, read from a book at night and save the tablets for daytime.

Late-night eating may disturb sleep. If our stomach has food to digest, then our body has to give attention and energy to that digestion. This may interrupt sleep.

Turn out the lights, turn down the temperature, and turn down the noise.

Try an aromatherapy infuser with a calming oil such as lavender to lull you to sleep. Dr. K struggles with getting in sleep due to early morning (5:00 a.m.) clients, but has found lavender fragrance in the bedroom helps her get a very restful night's sleep.

Wake up and remember this tidbit. Researchers have identified a toxic protein, amyloid, which builds up plaque in the brain when we have disrupted sleep, that is associated with Alzheimer's disease. They are not certain if the buildup leads to poor sleep or if poor sleep leads to a buildup of plaque.

TRAIN YOUR BRAIN WITH COGNITIVE EXERCISE

Everyone is talking about cognitive decline, cognitive function, cognitive improvements. What's the big interest? Well, an ever-growing and aging population and a malady that affects millions (see statistics below) at a cost that is difficult to put a price tag on should concern us all. Cognitive decline leads to a slew of poor health outcomes and quality of life. Exercise has been demonstrated to provide a generalized effect in improving cognitive functions such as:

- Speed of info processing
- Spatial abilities
- Executive functions
  - Critical thinking
  - Long-range thinking
  - Problem solving
- Attention
  - Receptive: measures the ability to focus and then shift attention between different stimulus under time pressure.
  - Expressive: measures attention selectivity and interference control under time pressure.

Exercise participation stimulates the growth of neurons (neurogenesis) in the hippocampus.

That's not a camp for hippos. The hippocampus, a small area within the center of the brain, is responsible for:

- Consolidation of new memories
- Emotional responses
- Navigation
- Spatial orientation

Studies in both human and nonhuman (mice) subjects have shown that exercise has a positive impact on learning and memory, spatial–navigational awareness, reaction time, mood, self-cognitions–self-perceptions, as well as general health benefits. It is a magic pill!

Some "food" for thought: US statistics on cognitive functioning and self-reported memory loss or confusion:

- age 45 and older = 12.5%**
- age 60 and older = 12.7% and 35% with functional difficulties*

Data Source: CDC Behavioral Risk Factor Surveillance System 2011* and 2012**

MAKE YOUR OWN "HAPPY PLACE"

To paraphrase John Mellencamp, "Dr. K was born in a small town, and Dr. K. lives in a small town, Dr. K. probably will die in a small town, and that is just fine by her." In fact, Dr. K lives in that same small town Mellencamp was singing about, Seymour, Indiana. She is unapologetically a "country girl," though more of the shabby chic variety than the trailer park type.

At any rate, I do have a big yard with lots of flowers and a couple of great outdoor spaces—a screened-in porch and a private patio off my bedroom. These are my in-town happy places. See, I like green things, things that grow, and during the warm months, these places have my houseplants on their summer vacation and some potted garden plants and herbs. This year I have three tomato plants, a zucchini, summer squash, and a cucumber. All are doing great and I will be picking soon.

I need space like this, so I created it. What kind of space do you need? List your space needs and then list what you need to create that space.

For me:

What I Want in Happy Place	Things Needed
Things that grow	Flowers, veggies/fruits
Birds	Birdfeeders/birdbaths
Pleasant outdoor sounds	Wind chimes, water fall/fountain
Place to sit or snooze	Hammock, chaise

CLUTTER-FREE LIVING

I am meticulous about the pictures on my wall being straight, the throw rugs being neat—however, look at the pile of mail and papers and you'd think—clean that crap up. Exactly! Well that said, keeping your home organized is a job in itself, and not a very fun job. So, work smarter, not harder.

- Keep mail in check by going through it before you sit it down.
- Put the junk mail, flyers, etc., directly into the recycle bin.
- File bills in a specific location, a desk tray or folder designated "bills."
  - Take it a step further and go to an office supply store and buy a dated file folder.
  - Place bills in folder 10 days prior to due date.

Chef D loves the look of midcentury modern art and design. The open format and clean lines have more than a touch of post–World War II Asian influence. For him it brings calmness to the living space and encourages clean all-American wholesome living. Think of it as feng shui meets Doris Day.

MyTendWell CHALLENGE

Create Compost

Repurposing furniture, clothes, barn wood . . . it's all the rage. Well, don't stop there, repurpose your food scraps, peels, and pits. And don't forget your yard clippings, trimmings, and cuttings to start a smart environmental wellness mission—keeping your organic waste out of the trash bags and ultimately the landfills. The combination of organic materials such as grass-clippings and fruit/veggie scraps will decompose into rich and fertile soil that can be added to your flower and garden beds.

Getting Started:

1. Purchase a countertop or floor container that tackles small amounts of refuse. Great for apartment and urban dwellers.

2. Find a space in a corner of your property in a sunny spot, that drains well and build bins out of land timbers, concrete blocks/ pavers/bricks. Fill bin with organic refuse such as:

   - Tree, grass clippings

   - Fruit and vegetable peels, pits and skins

   - Manure (Dr. K uses some of her horse manure to give the mix a little extra punch. Do not use dog or cat feces as these contain bacteria from meat digestion; farm animal manure is fine.)

INDOOR HOUSEPLANTS

Add some little green friends to your life and home. Not Martians, just some cheery houseplants. A few green leafy friends help "oxygenate" your home and bring some green indoors. The color green has been associated with stimulating the production of oxytocin—not OxyContin—better! It's the natural feel-good hormone. Mothers experience this effect when they look at their new babies as they nurse them. It's associated with romantic feelings, too! So, fall in love with some Philodendron.

Chef D and Dr. K's Top Five Houseplants

#1—Aloe Vera

Aloe gel has a number of healing properties. As most know, aloe is great for burns—from both the sun and touching hot stuff. It is also good for softening dry and cracked skin. Just break off a leaf and rub the gel onto your skin. Aloe is great for home air quality—clearing pollutants. It may also display brown spots if the air quality gets bad. Aloe grows best with lots of sun.

#2—Philodendron

See—Phil—odendron is a romantic, with its heart-shaped leaves, and clearly so loved. Where don't you see a Philodendron? It is a popular plant for indoors as they're easy to care for, grow decorative vines, and last for many years. Grow them with moderate water and some sunlight— Philodendron are good at absorbing xylene.

#3—Spider Plant

Most of us have an aversion to those eight-legged spiders that crawl across the floor, but spider plants are very popular. Spider plants are attractive and easy to grow. NASA counts spider plants on its list of the best air-purifying plants—effective at eliminating pollutants such as benzene, formaldehyde, carbon monoxide, and xylene.

#4—Golden Pothos

Optimal lighting to grow houseplants can be challenging; it seems like most need bright sunlight. The golden pothos is different: it does well in low light and will grow nice vines that add some drama to a corner of the room. Our #4 also is on the NASA list for cleaning formaldehyde out of the air.

#5—Peace Lily

This blooming beauty is a nice addition to your home—sending up shoots of peaceful blooms. The peace lily is low maintenance and does well in shade and cooler temperatures. The peace lily is also good at reducing toxins in the air.

BUILDING HEALTHY SOCIAL NETWORKS

Social engagement is a big topic in research on aging. The importance of staying connected as we age is important to our quality of life. Friends and confidants provide our social support network. As families grow up and move away and elder members die, our family network shrinks. Rebuild your family with friends—be each other's sisters and brothers in aging. Our evolutionary path consisted of social networks. Brain expansion theorists suggest that the large number of social contacts contributed to our early brain-size increase. Those social contacts are important, and as we age, we need that support system. Tend to your social wellness by scheduling buddy time with those friends.

Chef D's advice to those with their nose to the grindstone: The restaurant biz offers its fair share of unhealthy social opportunities. We are often working when everyone else is playing and playing when everyone else is sleeping. It is important that you separate your work life from your social life. It is tempting you to go to the local "chef's bar" and hang out with folks from the industry, but you might find yourself

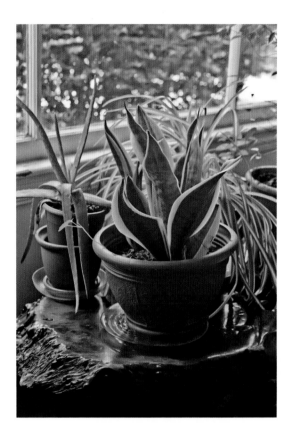

unfulfilled at the end of the day. Try following your passions. Take a pottery or painting class. Join a sports team. Take up golf; you can play that by yourself and still meet new people. The point is, take a step outside the box and put yourself somewhere you can rub elbows with someone other than a sweaty line cook or disgruntled server.

MOVEMENT BASICS

Basic **A**lignment for **C**ore and **K**inesthetic **S**tability (**B·A·C·K·S·**)

Movement. I've been fascinated with movement since I was a child. I watched the way people would walk, lift, carry, sit, and climb . . . MOVE. It truly fascinated me as I would watch the way my grandfather would carry feed to the cows, or the way my grandmother would plant the garden with her foot. Yes, her foot—true

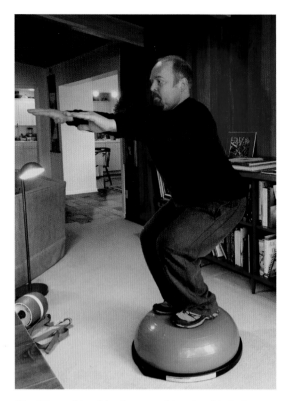

Chef D working his glutes and honing his balance on his BOSU.

CARING FOR OTHERS

As we age, so do those around us, including our parents, and most of my clients care for their parents, people in their 80s and 90s. This is a challenge—physically, emotionally, and financially. It's tough. But you need to do it, so prepare now. Begin getting yourself physically fit to have the energy and strength to give care to your loved ones.

Dr. K's Quick Tip: Practice Sit-to-Stands—training for daily living. This movement will keep you getting up and down—from a chair or from the toilet.

plantar flexion. She would make a hole with her big toe, drop in a seed and cover it with her foot. I was amazed and still not able to do as she could. When I watch sports competitions, I'm usually just watching the athletes execute their tasks—that is, move. Thus my gravitation to degrees and careers in kinesiology isn't surprising. Yes, kinesiology, the study of human movement.

My interest in human movement has led me to work within various roles, from fitness instructor/trainer to researcher of human positional behaviors. Ultimately I am interested in how people move, and I like to help people move better: from improving gait mechanics to enhancing how people execute their work tasks. I enjoy teaching people how to move better by educating them about how their bodies are currently moving and suggest tweaking if needed. I teach people to consider the environment in which they live and function and how their bodies interface with that environment. Regardless of the individuals and their environments, I always teach my clients B.A.C.K.S. Learning this technique of movement control is the essential ingredient to moving efficiently. This is what I call the ABC's of movement.

Just as a Chef D and his kitchen staff begin their days with prep and mise en place, so should we all. Aptly applied, prep and mise in this inference pertains to the ABC's of establishing and maintaining B.A.C.K.S. so that you are physically ready to begin and function throughout your day.

Follow this recipe and you will have the basics for creating an efficient body.

THE B.A.C.K.S. RECIPE: A+B+C = E (EFFICIENCY)—THE INGREDIENTS

A = Alignment: To maintain proper postural alignment (anatomically correct position), you should work to achieve and maintain the following positional alignment protocol by aligning the joints in the following checklist:

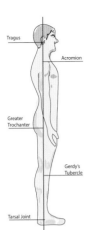

- Ears over shoulders
- Shoulders over hips
- Hips over knees
- Knees over ankles

Think of a carpenter's plumb line that runs through this positional alignment protocol, then work to maintain this alignment throughout the day and during all tasks you perform.

B = Balance: Balance has many meanings and connotations associated with health and wellness. First, maintaining good static (stationary) and dynamic (motion) balance is essential to health and well-being and requires that one establish and maintain the above proper postural alignment. Further, in order to establish and maintain balance, it is necessary to have appropriate muscle balance, that is, opposing muscle groups should have appropriate range of motion (flexibility), as well as appropriate strength. Importantly, good muscle and joint health and postural balance decrease the risk of injury and of falls. Ideally, we all should start moving from the perspective that we are moving with *purpose* toward a *goal*. That is, to improve functional capacity, to age successfully, and to avoid a *health apocalypse*.

C = Control: The utilization of good motor control during movement execution, from controlling static positional behaviors to controlling dynamic positional behaviors, is essential for movement efficiency. Our bodies evolved as a response to the environment in which we lived. The modern human form has movement capabilities as well as limitations. First, learning your own body's capabilities and limitations is important. Second, learning to utilize kinesthetic information, such as proprioception, and to adjust and correct posture and movement with consideration of your body's capabilities and limitations, prepares you to maintain motor control.

Balance—with meals, with activity, with friends and family—LIFE! Balancing out all the tasks that you need to do with all the things you want to do—it is a balancing act. Find a life balance that is rewarding for you and your loved ones. Plan your week so you've balanced your meals, movement, and mates.

Once you've got a plan for a well-balanced life, you will also want to be certain you've included balance training—for navigating through the courses of life.

Balance training can be as simple as creating a navigation course on your frequent hikes. My hiking mate, Ellen, and I have hiked from the Rockies of Colorado to the Knobs of Indiana—it's all good, but we like to step up our hiking game. We have a few regular hiking trails, so we use logs, rocks, and even tree roots as balance course obstacles. Instead of walking past that log, try walking along it. Try hopping from an exposed tree root to an exposed rock. Just be smart. Start small and simple, and build your balance skills. Yes, skills—and it takes practice. It's a great way to kick-up your hike.

> Dr. K also uses berry picking as a balance workout—nothing like reaching into a briar patch for sweet berries . . . and not falling in!

E = Energy: It takes energy to create energy. I could go on and on, provide chemical equations, discuss the processes of how we use energy to get energy from those precious resources (the metabolic cost of digestion) we pursue, but Chef D and I want you to understand relevance and

> My energy was gone after cancer. I used to be like the energizer bunny! I'd turn the music on and put my mic on, and I was on. I would teach two classes a day, coach clients, and keep up with my little boys, house, and garden/yard. I was a powerhouse of vigor (an important trait in health research). After cancer, I had no pep to my step (walking speed linked to longevity). I puttered around, draggin' ass. I had to get back to the ole me. Persistence with the MyTendWell Lifestyle Plan is what saved my ass: better, regular nutrition, better sleep, and more movement.
>
> It does take energy (that impetus, motivation) to create energy. But you have to be persistent—DAILY movement that keeps you strong and mobile.

application ideas. So, simply put, you have to invest a little (energy) on the front end in order to get a payout (energy) on the back end, so to speak. For many people, trying to fit physical activity into the day is a challenge that many do not meet due to a (perceived) *lack of time*. Research has identified that adherence to physical activity and exercise programs is about 50 percent. In other words, if I start an 8-week, 2x/week exercise class and 12 people sign up, at the end of that scheduled time, 6 people will be actively participating. The other half? They didn't stick, and the number one reason? *Perceived lack of time*. Yes. Perceived. Most likely the time was there, but the follow-through to participate and the commitment was not. Why? Well, if we are going to discuss "why" people do and do not do something, let's clear the table and address a very important point—exercise behavior is not a small nutshell that is easy to crack. In fact, it is a bunch of different nutshells that are tough to crack—it's called human behavior. So, to identify a single reason as to why people do not

participate in regular physical activity or exercise is not plausible. However, when people are asked about participation adherence, time *is* the number one reason. However, it is perceived lack of time. People are always willing to take the time to do the things they really want to do, the things they truly *enjoy*. **ENJOY**. That is key. In fact, organizations have added *Enjoyment* to exercise prescriptions such as with **FITTE** principles in which **F** is for *Frequency*, **I** is for *Intensity*, **T** is for *Type* (mode), **T** is for *Time*, and **E** is for *Enjoyment* and was only recently included (the original acronym was FITT). Researchers and practitioners have recognized that enjoyment is necessary and is important in getting people to stick with a physical activity/exercise program. I have worked with numerous individuals and groups in physical activity/exercise–based programs. People are more likely to continue if they enjoy what they are doing. Therefore, Chef D and I have created a wellness program that is enjoyable: a program that you will want to continue with in order to achieve the benefits of persistent physical activity. And one of those benefits is more energy. But in order to achieve that benefit, you must *make the time* to participate and you will gain more energy. So, now is the *time* to put a little energy in to get a little more energy out. Put down this book and take a 10-minute walk. Enjoy walking around your neighborhood. Maybe go to a local park; take a friend and find the enjoyment in movement. This energy will be the new skip to your step; your own internally driven boost.

Core Cinch: Just as a head of cabbage has its core, and the earth has its core, so too do we. Our core, our center, is the point from which all of our movement is anchored. Think of your core as the anchor that provides the foundation for the movements that we perform each and every day. In other words, *let the dog (core) wag the tail (limbs), not the tail (limbs) wag the dog (core)*. If you execute your tasks, from doing sit-to-stands, to walking, especially walking, you will find that you are moving more efficiently, simply due to moving your body in the biomechanical way it is designed to move. Further, by keeping your core strong and stable, you will decrease your risk of back injury as well as decrease pain and discomfort. Back pain is one of the top reasons for doctors' visits and afflicts individuals in all job tasks, from prolonged sitting and standing to trunk rotation.

Many of the repeated and prolonged postures we assume in our daily lives contribute to problems of the musculoskeletal system, such as low-back pain, for instance. Sedentary postures present an increased risk for musculoskeletal disorders (MSDs) such as chronic pain or

---

RECIPE FOR A HEALTHY SPINE

Core Cinch =

- Draw navel inward toward the spine and upward toward the ribs

- Draw your shoulder blades inward toward the spine and downward toward the hips.

Use this movement to stabilize and support the spine during all tasks— sitting, lifting—ALL movement!

---

discomfort in the joints of the neck, shoulder, wrists, hips, knees, and, most commonly, the back. Prolonged seated postures create a confined or constrained posture, which increases the risk of muscle fatigue brought on by low levels of muscle force for long periods of time in addition to restricted blood flow into and out of tissue. When in a seated posture, it is likely the pelvis will tilt posteriorly, decreasing the lordosis of the lumbar vertebra and consequently increasing the lumbar disk pressure. These confined postures limit blood flow into soft tissues, thus decreasing the flow of oxygenated blood and allowing for the buildup of metabolites. Essentially, there is no ideal prolonged posture,

and muscle fatigue can occur due to the low levels of muscle loading and decrease in blood flow. In order to decrease these risks, it is necessary to allow for frequent changes or variations in working postures—or simply put, make time for stretching/muscle lengthening and maintain good musculoskeletal health, especially improving muscle endurance of the postural stabilizers.

Common Concerns for the Back:

- Sedentary postures contribute to an increased risk of disk herniation.

- Too much or too little sitting or standing contribute to an increased risk of back pain.

- Prolonged, seated postures aggravate back pain and discomfort in individuals with ongoing symptoms.

- Bending and twisting motions are significantly related to low-back pain.

Common Concerns for the Neck and Shoulders:

- Working in bent or twisted postures contributes to an increased risk of neck and shoulder pain (e.g., for dental professionals, such as my big sis).

- Working with arms in unsupported forward flexion, such as in using a keyboard, contributes to pain and discomfort of neck and shoulders.

Quick Tip: Dr. K recommends following a DAILY program of physical activity that includes muscle strengthening, range-of-motion (flexibility) exercises, and balance training by incorporating the Fab Five from below.

Quick Tip: Dr. K suggests that you break up long periods of sitting with some stretching, which can be done at your desk. If you want to mix up your seated posture, try using a stability ball in place of your chair.

The MyTendWell Plan: Fab Five

"Core-the-cabbage"/ "Core Cinch"
Draw navel inward and upward and shoulder blades inward and downward. Do all day, every day. Ears over shoulders, shoulders over hips, hips over knees, knees over ankles—to align and maintain a neutral spine.

"Stir-the-Pot" Using the pot scrubber do circular motions with each leg rotating the ball joint in your hip sideways.

"Dip-the-Hip" Move the leg forward using the pot scrubber while dipping with the opposite thigh. Keep core under control.

"The Rotisserie Funky Chicken"
Act like a football ref giving the field goal sign. Rotate the shoulders by moving the arms up and down.

"Tilt-the-Skillet" From a seated position, hinge forward from the hip, keep spine-in-align, and hinge back up to a seated position.

GETTING REAL WITH THE SMART GOAL SHEET AND LOG BOOK: A NUTRITION AND PHYSICAL ACTIVITY LOGBOOK/APP

Before you start your new regime, we suggest you keep a food and movement journal for at least three days. Eat what you normally do, but just write it down. Same with activity, write it all down. If you have ever wondered why you put on weight, it will quickly become evident. People who do this will generally start modifying their food intake because the facts show up in black and white. There is no disputing it. Remember to be honest. This is for you and being inaccurate will only be cheating yourself. If you aren't honest, you won't have the fun of realizing real change! Nutrition and activity journals are extremely helpful for your doctor, nutritionist, and wellness coaches, so take your journals with you on your next appointment. Ask the professionals for advice as well. You can go to our website, www.mytendwell.com, and download the forms, and keep them in a folder or simply transfer the information to a similar format. Chef D likes to fold the page up and keep it in his pocket so he can make notes on it all day. Make sure you write all the foods down as you eat them and all your activity. You'd be amazed how quickly you can forget what you ate 30 minutes ago. Heck, 2 minutes ago.

Who Sticks and Who Quits?

Being enticed or tempted is a serious challenge and a deterrent to maintaining or sticking to a healthy behavior, whether it is your physical activity plan or your nutrition plan. Having accountability assists with keeping on track. Using the MyTendWell Lifestyle Plan Activity and Nutrition Log provides a place to track your behavior and share with someone (see website). This will help you become accountable and help you stick to your plan for achieving your goal.

Look, adherence to physical activity, at best, is 50 percent. Further, in spite of all the developments—interventions and programs, facilities, equipment and products—no impact has been made on improving adherence to physical activity/exercise behavior since it was first tracked in the early 1900s at Springfield College. Simply put, only half stick, the rest fall to the wayside. So, as practitioners and researchers alike, we want to know why. Why do people stick? Why do people quit?

Why do people stick (adhere)?

- Self-motivation
- Social support
- Goal setting (having a plan)

The MyTendWell Lifestyle Plan Movement Toolbox

Top Five Movement Tools

In order to reach those movement goals, you have to stick to the MyTendWell Lifestyle Plan. Remember: *Persistent application toward one steadfast goal.* Persistence! This is a lifestyle you are adopting. It's not a sprint but an endurance event, so you have to find ways to keep active by being proactive. This is how to set yourself up for success.

Dr. K knows that access to movement options is necessary for individual wellness success and has created the MyTendWell Lifestyle Plan Movement Toolbox so you can have access to movement tools at home, work or travel.

1. **Resistance Tubing:** Just a couple of resistance tubes and you have a weight set for home, work, and travel. There is an array of options so buy a few of varying resistance and you'll be able to strength train all your muscles.

2. **Stretch Strap:** Again, there is an array of options, so buy what you like. This item will help improve range of motion (flexibility) in your most troublesome areas.

3. **Pot Scrubbers:** Large plastic-bottomed furniture movers for destabilization exercises. You'll love this durable and portable balance trainer. They usually come in a pack of four, so buy a set and share with a friend. A gift that keeps on giving.

4. **Foam Mat:** You'll want to protect that spine when doing core work, so get a mat that has a bit of foam cushion. Most roll up and come with a handy strap that makes it portable.

5. **Stability Ball:** A great tool that has been used for decades and is adaptable for a lot of uses, from exercise tool to modified office chair. (Learn more about Dr. K's research on stability ball use as an intervention for sedentary behavior at www.mytendwell.com).

Additional item: Canvas or mesh bag for storing and transporting resistance tubes, stretch strap, and pot scrubbers.

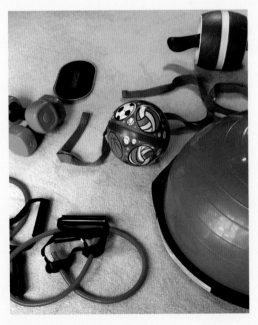

Dr. K.'s workout "toolbox."

Why do people quit?

- Time (perceived lack of time)
- Access to facility/space (indoor/outdoor recreation area, sidewalks)
- Lack of knowledge/instruction—poor education in health and wellness

MyTendWell Lifestyle Plan considers these factors and requires individuals set SMART Goals. This is how Dr. K helped Chef D. He had to set SMART Goals, identify barriers, create a Toolbox, build his environment to support physical activity, and log every day. There have been ups and downs, but Chef D has learned a lot about himself along the way. So, if you are wondering if Chef D is motivated to be physically active, the answer is yes. What does Chef D like? Deep Water Exercise. His biggest barrier: Time and access.

The MyTendWell Lifestyle Plan: Back-in-Five Movement Breaks

Energy wanes as we sit. Why wouldn't it? Our body "thinks" we are on shut-down mode–physiologic rest, so to speak. Remind your body you are awake with a take five movement break.

Dr. K's Back-in-Five

Desk jockeys, long-distance haulers—too much sitting is not a good thing, nor is too much standing. Break up those static, prolonged behaviors with a Take Five (minutes) Movement Break:

1. Three-minute brisk walk
2. 10–15 Dip-the-Hip
3. 10–15 Rotisserie Funky Chicken
4. 10–15 Tilt-the-Skillet
5. Five deep breathes in through the nose and out through the mouth
6. Feel refreshed.

HOW DOES GOAL SETTING ASSIST IN REACHING GOALS?

1. Directing activity
2. Mobilizing effort
3. Increasing persistence
4. Motivating the search for appropriate strategies

WHAT IS A MyTendWell LIFESTYLE PLAN SMART GOAL?

We are all familiar with the saying "Keep your eyes on the prize." Well, that's code for stick to your goal. There is a reason you are interested in the MyTendWell Lifestyle Plan: you have a goal and you want to reach it, and goal setting is important in reaching goals. The trick is to set a *specific goal*. A goal that is measurable, a goal that is attainable and realistic. And a goal that can be met in the time frame allotted.

Specific: Be explicit with your goal by stating it clearly. For example, I will do 30 minutes of brisk walking on Monday, Tuesday, Thursday, Friday, and Saturday. I will do 30 minutes of resistance training on Wednesday and Sunday.

Measurable: Identify a quantifiable goal. For example, 30 minutes of brisk walking on Monday, Tuesday, Thursday, Friday, and Saturday and 30 minutes of resistance training on Wednesday and Sunday.

Attainable: Set a goal that you can achieve. For example, if you are not a runner, instead of setting a goal of running a 5K, perhaps start with walking a 5K.

Realistic: Be logical with your goals. For example, if you are not a "morning person," setting a goal of working out in the morning may not be realistic. Instead, perhaps a noontime workout during the week and a midmorning on weekends.

Time frame: Be reasonable with the time frame in which you can complete your goal. For example, getting prepared to run a half-marathon takes a few months. Make certain your time frame is sensible.

MyTendWell CHALLENGE: Strategies for Behavioral Change

Identify your goals, set your timeline, and put your plan into action. Review Stages of Change in chapter 2. Adjust your environment to minimize barriers: to physical activity, to eating before bedtime, to spending quality time with love ones.

Some tips:

1. Identify the negative behavior (skipped sessions, shortened sessions, poor compliance to meal plans).

2. Identify stimuli/situations that lead to the negative behavior (stress, fatigue, snacking/poor meals).

3. Develop counterstrategies: For instance, special exercise sessions—energizing, stress buster workouts, recreation assignments.

Important points

Stimulus Control: Avoiding or managing stimuli that lead to inactivity.

Counterconditioning: Substituting alternatives for problem behaviors that foster inactivity or that lead to disordered eating.

The MyTendWell Lifestyle Plan: Five Steps to Cultivate your SMART Goal

1. Write your SMART goal for each dimension of the MyTendWell Plan.

2. Make a list of triggers and barriers.

3. Make a list of strategies to deal with trigger and barriers.

4. Journal in your MyTendWell log every day for your first 30 days (minimum).

   - Write down everything you eat. Be specific—include quantity.

   - Write down your physical activity/ exercise behavior.

   - Be sure to include all activity/ behavior that addresses any of the eight dimensions of wellness from the MyTendWell flower: social, occupational, intellectual, physical, emotional, spiritual, environmental, and nutritional.

5. Evaluate your progress. You may need to revise your plan.

   - Are you meeting your nutritional wellness goals? Yes/No

   - Are you meeting your physical wellness goals? Yes/No

   - Are you meeting your other wellness goals? Yes/No

   - Have you had an improvement in energy, sleep? Yes/No

   - Are you enjoying life more fully? Yes/No

Behavior change is dependent on your ability to learn about yourself and your environment. This requires attention and effort—be sure you give it your all!

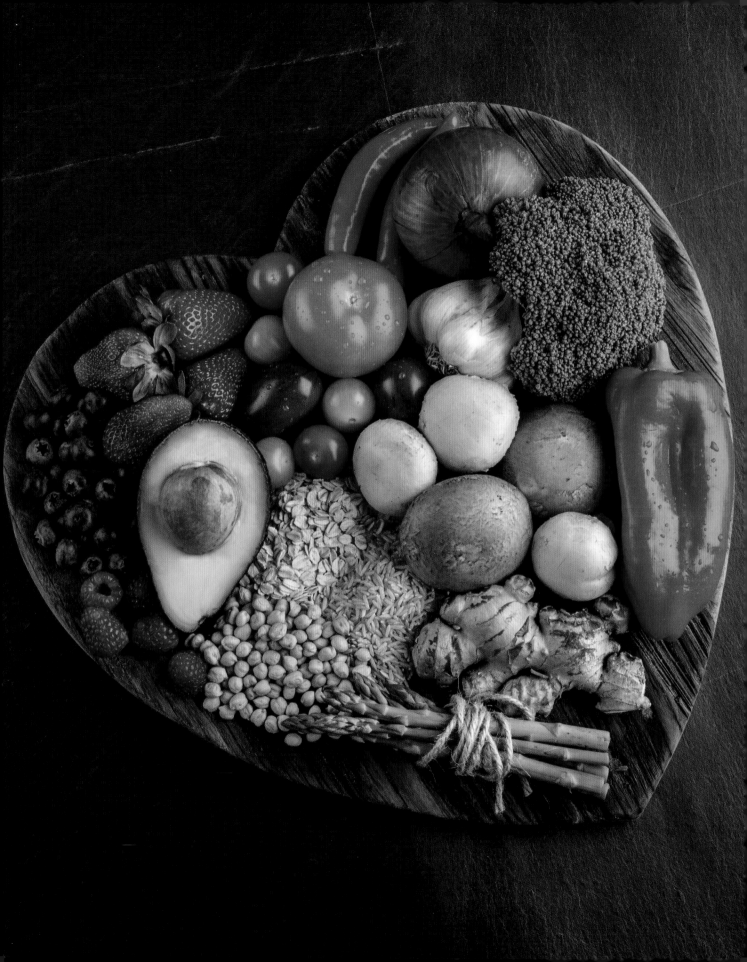

4

Enlightening Your Life

THE TREMENDOUS 20—MY SUPERHEROES IN THE KITCHEN

I was intrigued by the book *SuperFoodsRx;* I loved the concept of being able to eat as much as you want of certain natural products, basically without the fear of overeating. As long as you eat these foods without "polluting" them with unhealthy ingredients, the world's pantry is your oyster. You'll have to check out the book to get the details. I recommend it highly.

In my Tremendous 20, I use a rainbow of colorful, high-powered foods I hope you will enjoy. Remember—you must enjoy! That is the single most important part of any lasting healthy lifestyle plan. Without looking for pleasure at the table, you will usually end up giving up. These are my Superheroes of the food world and their sidekicks.

MY SUPERHEROES IN THE KITCHEN

Awesome Agua (a.k.a. water): Our bodies are made up mostly of water, so it only makes sense that water's essential! Water, like oil in a machine, keeps us lubricated and moving smoothly. It also provides many other benefits, such as washing away toxins and keeping us cool through perspiration. Good, pure water, and plenty of it, will keep skin looking young and fresh and assist in regulating body temperature and removing waste products, so it's important

to replace water lost after a good hard workout (i.e., workouts at the gym or in the work world). Water has zero calories and cleanses internal organs, keeping them flushed out and ready for the demands of their functions. Plain old steam-distilled water is the best. It is purified in the distilling process and is free of metallic tastes. If you prefer, and can afford, spring waters, there are many available, each with a unique flavor and mineral profile. There are also many fancy flavored "sports waters" out there with various additives, but if you eat a healthy diet you will already have taken care of your nutritional needs.

Water—the forgotten "nutrient"—is important in providing hydration, replacing water lost through urination, defecation, and perspiration. Maintaining proper hydration assists in temperature regulation as well as all chemical processes in the body.

Make your own flavored waters! They are cheaper and better for you. Just add slices of cucumber, fruit, citrus, or herbs to a pitcher of ice, bruise them by stirring, and top it all off with water. Add a great variety of delicious and healthy flavors to water for yourself and for your parties and get-togethers. Drink up the good life.

These are just an added expense. Stay away from sweetened water and waters with artificial additives. Waters are supposed to be natural. Drink water instead of sweetened drinks. Water, unlike fruit juice and soda, does not raise your insulin levels and is easily absorbed. So, if you are looking to hydrate, make a date with a tall glass of water!

Bodacious Berries: Chefs love berries. They make our lives easy. Almost any dessert looks better sprinkled with a few. Where would we be without raspberry coulis to paint our plates and make our mousses with? So it's nice to have these old friends on my shopping list. Berries are full of antioxidants as well as some of the same tannins that make red wine so good for us. Berries may be added to grain salads and blended into vinaigrettes. Blackberries and blueberries are both rich in anthocyanins and fiber. They are especially suggested for eye health, slowing macular degenerative disease.

> **Berries** are packed full of antioxidants—those wonderful substances that work to remove or interfere with free radicals, which cause oxidative stress. Oxidative stress to our "biological machine" may be a factor in the development of cancer. Foods rich in antioxidants include berries, coffee beans, herbs, and green tea.

Bangin' Broccoli: Broccoli and other cruciferous vegetables are full of vitamins and minerals as well as fiber. As an added bonus they are good for your skin! At least that is what my mom told me when I was a teenager. Maybe that was just her way of getting me to eat them. Cruciferous vegetables are members of the cabbage family including cauliflower, kale, Brussels sprouts, and kohlrabi. Scientists have found strong evidence that this family of vegetables may actually

be powerful in preventing cancer, particularly that of the stomach and colon. Tests in a breast cancer study showed that daily consumption lessened the risk by 24 percent compared to another test group eating only one serving every 10 days. Cruciferous vegetables contain chemicals that seem to change the effect of estrogen. These veggies are also high in vitamin K, so people on anticoagulants should check with doctors before changing their diets.

> **Broccoli** is loaded with phytochemicals that may have cancer-preventive properties. Studies have shown that people who ate approximately five servings of fruits and vegetables per day were half as likely to develop cancer as those who ate only two servings per day . . . so do eat your broccoli . . . it's a super veggie!

Big Bad Beans: Here's the stink on beans. They are legumes, which are members of the species of plants that includes beans, peas, and lentils. Legumes are a major low-fat source of minerals such as potassium, magnesium, and zinc; they also provide complex carbohydrates, protein, and fiber. Many cultures' diets, such as those of the Mayans and some Native Americans, were built around the combination of beans and corn (Indian corn or maize) for their protein source. People joke about getting a bit gassy from beans, but anytime you change your diet it is likely to take a little time for your body to adjust. Don't let this keep you from adding more beans to your diet. Your body will adjust in a week or two. Try beano®, an enzyme formula that breaks down the gas-forming part of the bean and other foods. Soaking beans in several changes of water and slow cooking them should help as well. The high amount of fiber contained in beans alerts you to drink plenty of water to help you usher them through!

> Many chronic diseases, including cancers, are thought to be caused by chronic inflammation. **Legumes or beans** include flavonoids, a class of polyphenols. Dietary polyphenol, investigated in animal models and epidemiological trials, may provide protective factors to reduce inflammatory mechanisms and assist in the prevention of certain cancers.

Chili-icious: For me, the most important quality of a chili is its flavor, although I love the heat and perfume of chilies as well. I remember walking down a dirt road in Belize and smelling the aroma of hot sauce being made. Every time I see a Scotch bonnet chili I think of it. Many cultures in hotter climates use chilies in their food as a cooling agent. The chilies make you sweat and as the sweat evaporates from your skin you are cooled. That is why they are used extensively in Vietnamese, Thai, Chinese, Mexican, Caribbean, and Indian dishes. I was shocked to find out they have so much nutritional value to them. A quarter cup of chilies has a vitamin C content of 91 milligrams! Even if you don't eat them by the bowlful, that is impressive. Choose red chilies and get a beta-carotene boost as well. All chilies start out green, but ripening increases their flavor and nutritional value. Capsaicin, the compound that gives chilies their lusty burn, seems to have a positive effect on blood cholesterol, and also works as an anticoagulant. Capsaicin's

> Research suggests that dietary practices can prevent nearly 35 percent of all cancers. Some of the food products in our regular diet are packed full of nutrients. **Capsaicin**, which is found in chili peppers, is just one of those food items that may inhibit tumor growth in cancers.

burn also is thought to raise your metabolism and help you burn more calories, thus making them a great diet food. "Chili Heads," people addicted to hot peppers, love the "high" they get from eating fiery chili-spiked foods. It is a natural drug that is both safe and legal. The endorphins sent to protect you from the pain create the sensation of pleasure.

Fabulous Fresh Herbs: Herbs can transform any bland and boring "healthy" dish into something to rave about. With the proper know-how you can cut back on fat and calories by using herbs in your cooking. A bit of chopped mint, dill, tarragon, or even plain old parsley bring freshness and life to many of Chef D's diet dishes. Herbs are easy to grow in the backyard, on a rooftop, or in a window box and are now available in most grocery stores. Herbs have the added benefit of containing more antioxidants than many fruits and vegetables. Fresh herbs contain large amounts of antioxidants like vitamin C, beta-carotene, and vitamin A. As little as a tablespoon of fresh herbs can beat the amount of antioxidants in an apple, so start thinking, "An HERB a day will keep the doctor away!" I'm sure Jack LaLanne would agree.

> Phytochemicals, capsaicinoids, and even the aromas and flavors of herbs and spices are associated with health benefits. The aromas of **herbs and spices** stimulate salivary processes, which, in turn, stimulate digestion. There are possible anticarcinogenic properties associated with phytochemicals in both herbs and spices.

Foraged Finds: Foraging is the act of hunting for wild varieties of vegetables and fruits in the great outdoors. To quote "Wildman" Steve Brill (Central Park's foraging guru), "Foraged produce is much more nutritious, and it's more fun to collect. These items are more nutritious because they have a greater concentration of nutrients. Commercial vegetables are bred to be heavier, to have more water and, consequently, less flavor and less nutrition. Wild plants also are free— and they're incredibly delicious. If you taste wild watercress and compare it to the watercress you buy in the store, for example, you'll never want the store-bought stuff again. Anyway, I'd rather go out picking in a nearby field than stand in line at the grocery store." Take Wildman's tour if you get to New York or buy a book on harvesting nature's bounty. It is a fun and healthy activity to do with family and friends. Just make sure you pick the right things.

> **Foraging** serves more than the purpose of finding unique and tasty treats in the woods or the backyard. It provides an opportunity to walk and to be in nature. Green exercise or activity in the outdoors has demonstrated a positive effect on mood. So, go out and forage, challenge your memory and spatial awareness. How well do you remember where you found those mushrooms last spring? Are you able to remember the clues that nature gives you, to direct you to new spots to find mushrooms?

Feeling Fruity: I often forget how tasty fresh fruit is. When I'm out at a restaurant I'm always tempted by something creamy, chocolaty, or caramely. But some of my most memorable eating experiences have to do with fruit. I still remember the taste of a perfectly ripe pear I ate fifteen years ago in front of a cathedral in the south of France, the juices of a ripe mango in the streets of Salvador, Bahia, Brazil, and the explosive flavor of the sun-warmed wild blackberries that grow across the street from my parents' Indiana home. Fruits come in a wide variety of flavors,

colors, textures, and sweetness. Always choose fruit that is picked at its ripest and shipped the shortest distance. I like to eat whole fruits on an empty stomach first thing in the morning. It gets the engine running and gets me fired up. It also seems to clear out the pipes and get me ready for a clean start. Many nutritionists suggest that you always eat fruit along with some sort of protein like a nut butter to slow the level of insulin brought about by the sugars in fruit. There has been a lot said about food combining and I suggest that you do your own research and make your own choices.

> **FINALLY!** US Nutrition Guidelines have upped their recommendations for fruit and veggies to 10 servings a day from 5. The fiber in fruits and veggies gets and keeps the pipes moving, and gastrointestinal motility is important. Letting your waste matter hang around in the intestines for too long increases risk of colon cancers and diverticulitis, causes you to feel uncomfortable, and makes a body grumpy.

Great Grains: Whole grains are cereals that contain all parts of the grain including the germ, endosperm, and outer bran layers. Most

> How about those wonderful complex carbohydrates? These rich in nutrients and high in fiber **whole grains** are great to build your diet around. Unlike the simple carbohydrates that metabolize quickly after spiking your blood sugar, complex carbohydrates break down more slowly, and therefore provide lower levels of sugars over a longer period of time . . . sustaining you with better fuel. Try to buy organic grains.

processed foods use only the starchy white endosperm. When purchasing prepared whole-grain foods make sure the predominant ingredient is whole grain. Fiber is helpful to all sorts of bodily functions and should be a large part of the human diet. It keeps us regular as well as keeps all our plumbing working properly. There are also plenty of those all-important antioxidants in whole grains. These include vitamin E and selenium, which are both good for skin and heart. Antioxidants slow down the formation of cataracts and other effects of the passage of time . . . a.k.a. aging.

> **Lycopene** is a carotenoid pigment and also a phytochemical. Lycopene has been investigated for its protective properties against cancer, especially breast cancer.

I See Red Tomatoes and other red vegetables: Tomatoes are often thought of as vegetables but they are more accurately berries. They contain high amounts of beta-carotene and the phytochemical lycopene. Tomatoes are known as nature's sunscreen because when eaten they are thought to help prevent sun damage from the inside out. Cooking tomatoes may reduce the amount of vitamins C and A but actually increases the amount of the lycopene, so a good balance of cooked and raw red veggies is required. Try red and orange peppers, too.

In a Nutshell: Nuts have a bad rap for being fatty. But theirs is good fat. As long as they are treated as a "controlled substance" (controlled by the eater!), they are extremely good for us. They are cholesterol-free and a good substitute for animal protein when combined with grains and vegetables. Nuts contain mono- or polyunsaturated fat, not the artery-clogging saturated fats. Nuts can even help reduce the nasty LDL cholesterol levels if eaten regularly in small quantities. Walnuts are full of linolenic acid, which can be converted to heart-healthy omega-3 fatty acids in the body. Almonds and pecans are other good options. Try some of the low-fat dairy replacements made from nuts such as almond cheese. These can be found in the health food and natural markets.

> **Nuts**, like chili peppers, provide some inhibitory factor in the growth of cancer cells. Nuts are packed with healthy fats, such as omega-3s, and are another good source of protein. Pack a snack with mixed nuts and dried fruit.

Lettuce Alone (the honeymoon salad): The nutritional value of lettuce varies with the variety. The more water content and lighter green color the less nutritious the lettuce. People who think they are doing themselves some good by chowing down on a wedge of iceberg with blue cheese and mayo dressing have another think coming to them. The good stuff is in the darker leaves of romaine, escarole, radicchio, and mâche. Lettuce is great when you start a diet because it gives you something crisp and crunchy to munch on without many calories. Most of the healthy fiber is in the ribs of the lettuce so don't cut those away.

Mean Greens: Dark green leafy vegetables have always been a staple of peasants, slaves, and farmers. They are relatively easy to grow and fulfill many of our dietary needs. Spinach, collards, mustard greens, and others all are full of vitamins A and C and folate. Spinach has tons of vitamin K that's great for building bone mass. Greens can be braised as a side dish, tossed in soups and stews, or used as a stuffing for fish or chicken. Simply sautéed with a little garlic and olive oil is my favorite way to serve them.

Oh My God, 3: No, it's not a movie sequel, it's a fat that we are allowed to eat! Omega-3 fatty acids are something people were afraid to talk about several years ago. Now people are eating as much wild salmon as they can get their hands on. Folks used to be afraid of fat, but fats are an important part of our diets. Just make sure you are balancing them properly and eating the right kinds. Healthy fats help us maintain good hair and skin, protect and insulate our bodies, transport vitamins and minerals throughout our bodies, and generally allow the body machine to function properly. Healthy fats are found in fish and seafood in high quantities but may also be found in avocados, flax seeds, purslane, free-range chicken eggs, and forest-raised natural pork.

> Packed full of antioxidant and micronutrients, **greens** are great for the diet and gut. Fibrous, leafy veggies add to GI (gastrointestinal) motility—keeping the pipes clean and happy.

Protein Power: Low-fat protein is an important part of every meal. Including it aids in digestion and increases our metabolism. This doesn't have to be animal protein; nuts, beans, low-fat dairy, and soy products are all good sources as well. Everyone knows that chicken and turkey breast have low-fat protein, but they also contain good amounts of B vitamins, potassium, iron, zinc, and phosphorus. I love the crispy poultry skin, but do push that to the side of the plate because it's the chicken fat! Begone, you chicken fat, begone! You may roast with the skin on to keep the

> **Omega-3 (linolenic acid) and omega-6 (linoleic acid)**, are considered essential fatty acids and are the only lipids (fats) required in our diet. These essential fatty acids are necessary in growth, reproduction, learning, vision, and bodily functions.

bird moist, but take it off after cooking (before slicing) to keep temptation away from the dinner table. Protein can be served in millions of ways but it still can get boring, so change things up by trying other low-fat sources. Fish, pork tenderloin, wild game, or the more expensive ostrich or buffalo are fun for experimenting. Also, try cooking tempeh and other vegetarian proteins.

> **Protein** is what a growing body needs. If you are doing strength training, and I'm sure you are, then you need those amino acids found in protein. These are the building blocks for maintaining and rebuilding healthy tissue—especially after injury or trauma such as surgery.

Soy, Oh Boy: Ancient Chinese secret, huh? I like to call tofu the scary white stuff. I've never seen grown men so frightened as when I mention that I will be preparing tofu in one of my cooking classes or demonstrations! But tofu is like a canvas, pale and welcoming, just waiting for you to be creative. Add colorful vegetables, sauces, and spices, and it soaks flavors up, becoming a piece of edible art. I like to make soy cream cheese, sour cream, and mayonnaise to add richness and low-fat protein to many of my recipes. There are many varieties of tofu, so try them all. They vary in texture more than flavor so use the silken varieties for sauces, shakes, and smoothies and the firmer ones for stir-fries, grilling, and salads. In many Asian markets, the tofu is displayed in open tubs of water. I suggest using this only for cooked recipes and always using packaged tofu for uncooked dishes and drinks. Try making your favorite chicken salad or tuna salad recipe with well-squeezed firm tofu and tofu mayo. Make un-deviled eggs by discarding the yolks and filling the eggs with a soy salad touched with curry to give the yellow color. Tofu may have once been an ancient secret outside

China, but today everyone is learning the joys of this simple ingredient.

> **Soy** products have demonstrated to be protective against some cancers, including breast cancer. Soy products are often high in sodium, so be aware.

Seductive Spices: Spices, like the fresh herbs above, give us flavor without fat. Freshly ground, they are like perfumes that when used properly can coax and highlight the flavors in all our foods. There are a huge number of spices from all around the world and discovering them and their cultural background is an exciting part of cooking healthy. Spices are like aphrodisiacs. Their flavors and aromas stimulate more than just taste buds. Use spices well and you might get lucky tonight. I love blending spices and offer you a variety online at **www.farm-bloomington.com**.

> **Spices** have essential oils that have antimicrobial and anticancer properties. Spices are also great substitutes for salt, adding flavorings salt alone can't achieve.

Sacred Squash: Winter squash was one of the first vegetables grown by the Native Americans. Their diet was based on the "Three Sisters": squash, corn, and beans. Winter squash, so called because of its ability to be stored for a long period of time, is high in beta carotene, which actually increases during storage. Winter squash is an excellent source of energy because it is low in fat, rich in potassium, and high in complex carbohydrates. Squash can be used in many creative ways in your kitchen. Try roasting, sautéing, and grilling for quick and easy meals or turning it into soups, sauces, and gratins when you have a few extra minutes.

> **Beta-carotene** is beneficial in the prevention of cataracts, cardiovascular disease, and cancer. It is found in carrots, sweet potatoes, mangoes, broccoli, kale, pumpkin, and many more delicious fruits and vegetables.

Sweet Citrus: All parts of the citrus fruit are important to our bodies, and whenever you are eating citrus you should remember this. If you do what I used to do, you chug orange juice right out of the box, standing in your underwear in front of the refrigerator first thing in the morning. Well, that isn't the best way to get the most out of citrus. What you do get that way is a huge sugar rush. You are much better off eating citrus sections so you get the important fiber that slows down digestion and allows you to get more nutrients from the fruit. Citrus's vitamins A and C may reduce the risk of some forms of cancer and help the body repair tissues. Folic acid has a role in preventing birth defects, heart disease, and some cancers. Potassium balances the fluids in our bodies and strengthens cell structure. Citrus fruits contain limonoids, carotenoids, and flavonoids, which new research now explains as important and necessary in a healthy diet. Pink grapefruit and blood oranges are particularly good for you.

> **Phytochemicals** are in many of the foods MyTendWell encourages adherents of the plan to add to their diets. These nutrients are associated with prevention of cancer, so peel a red grapefruit—no need to slice and sweeten with sugar.

Yo Gurty!: This old girl has been with us since about 5,000 BCE. Humans have known about yogurt longer than they've known about religion! Although the nutritional value is much like that of milk, there is a nice richness to yogurt that makes it a perfect replacement for the fattier dairy products like cream, sour cream, and whole milk. You can even drain off the whey (the thin, watery liquid, perfect to reserve and add to your morning smoothie) and you'll have a rich soft cheese called labne. Streptococcus thermophilus and Lactobacillus bulgaricus are the bacteria used in turning milk to yogurt, but don't be scared of their names. They are important and naturally occur in our intestines. Yogurt can be used to reintroduce natural flora to your diges-

> **Yogurt** is another way of getting protein in the morning. Mornings can be a rush, so have a cup of yogurt, top it with fresh fruit, nuts, some flax seed, or wheat germ. By mixing the protein with the natural sugars in fruit and fibers of whole grains, this breakfast will pack a punch of energy for hours. Check out the strained Greek varieties. Yummy!

tive tract after you've taken strong antibiotics. Many lactose-intolerant children and adults can eat yogurt and yogurt products, which are great calcium sources. Yogurt has been a dietary staple for generations of Russian mountain people, many of whom live to be 100! So, eat it and eat it often.

HOW TO TRULY ENJOY YOUR FOOD

You chew and swallow, right? Well, those are the basics, but there is really much more to it than that . . . how far do you want to take it? My passion led me to cooking school, to cooking and eating through America, Europe, and Central and South America, to running a 700-seat

MyTendWell CHALLENGE

Now that you've learned what the evil empire consists of and how to overthrow it with the Tremendous 20, Chef D and Dr. K challenge you to take up these weapons of body mass reconstruction, defeat your food enemies, and regain your health. Use the MyTendWell Activity and Nutrition Log found at **mytendwell.com** to record your food and movement—everyday! Track changes in your energy, mood, and even, don't forget, the happenings from your porcelain throne. In other words, pay attention to how the changes in your diet and movement change your "deposits." Changes in your diet (limiting white sugar and white flour) and changes in your movement behavior (moving at least 30 minutes every day) will change your fecal matter. Adding whole-grain fibers, increasing water intake, as well as stimulating the gastrointestinal (GI) track with physical movement will impact your bowel movements—in a positive way. Bowel movements should be solid and regular. Track your changes; after one week, you will notice the difference.

complex of restaurants, bars, and private rooms, and to cooking in paradise on a Caribbean isle. Enjoying food can truly be a way of life; in fact, it can take over your life! Having a passion for food is great; having a compulsion about it is another story. This is coming from a guy who owns over a thousand cookbooks, so many I have to put half of them in storage. Is that just plain crazy?

I always thought I was enjoying food, but it took dealing with a 40-pound weight gain to make me question if I really knew what appreciation of food is all about. At first I was pissed

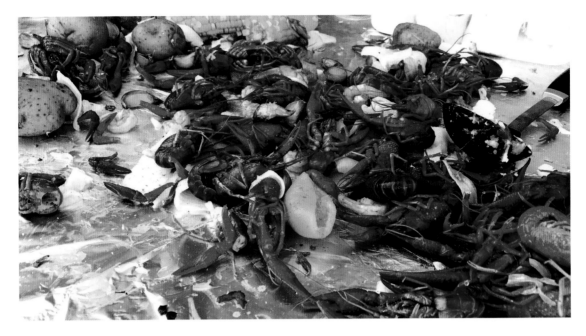

off that I had to curb my enthusiasm at the dinner table, but I soon learned that to enjoy life, I would have to think deeper than my taste buds. Food can have too much emotion tied to it. If your body isn't dealing with your food in a healthy way, giving you energy and a spring in your step, then you need to learn how to better choose your foods.

I found that keeping a journal of everything that went in my mouth and the timing of eating was a very telling tale. It is like keeping a diary wherein you tell all your secrets. Believe me, if you're honest with yourself, it won't take you long to understand what you are doing wrong and accept that a change is needed. Once you've done this for a week or two, see how it matches up with the MyTendWell Lifestyle Plan and make the appropriate changes. You will be amazed how quickly you begin to feel more energetic and clearheaded, and this realization will bring you more joy than the brief satisfaction those chips deliver. Once you've set your new path you will enjoy the additional foods, flavors, and textures that come into your life. Tofu will no longer be the "scary white stuff" if you turn it into sour cream, cream cheese, or mayonnaise. Sprouts and nuts won't be boring if they are sprinkled

over a spicy avocado soup. Burdock, salsify, and sunchokes won't be strangers when you make them into a crispy salad that will blow that old picnic potato salad away.

To truly enjoy food takes some thinking, planning, and passion. You must use all your senses. Of course you touch the food when you are shopping and cooking, but I also love dishes that you pick up when you are eating. Shell-on shrimp, artichokes, and corn on the cob are all great because you have to slow down and savor them, not just shovel them into your mouth. Touching food has much more to it than finger touching; it also has to do with the way food feels in the mouth. Smooth and creamy or crunchy or chewy all have to do with the way food touches you on the inside of your mouth. Smelling food is a given; many say that aroma is 50 percent of tasting. What might not be as evident is that smelling can also save you from disaster. I smell oysters before I serve or eat them and always do a nose check before tasting if I have a question about how long something has been in the fridge. People eat with their eyes; everyone knows that, but a smile from the ones with whom you share food makes things taste even better. Tasting is the sensation you have when food or drinks

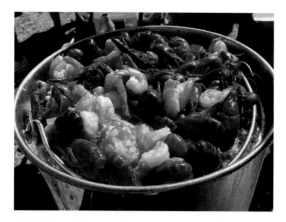
Trio of crayfish.

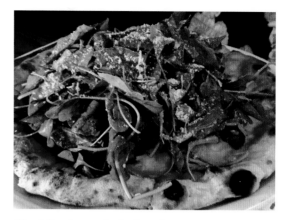
Wood-fired arugula flatbread.

dance on your taste buds. Take the time to notice how things taste throughout their journey through your mouth. There is a start, a middle, and a finish, and chefs are trying to make each area sing. When in restaurants or at the home of a great cook, take time to appraise and appreciate a dish on the first couple of bites; then do the same with the addition of wine. Notice sweet, bitter, sour, acid, saline, fatty, spice, and herbal flavors and think about how you can take those ideas home and include them in your own wonderfully nutritious meals. And, believe it or not, hearing is also part of cooking. Listening to vegetables sizzling in olive oil lets you know they are doing their thing. You can even hear water coming to a boil, but, beyond that, you can hear the praise of your loving friends and family for a job well done. I'd better mention the sound of the fire alarm going off when you've left something in the oven too long.

Truly enjoying food means taking the time to cook a fully satisfying meal or finding a restaurant that serves inspiring healthy and tasty cuisine. But that is just the start. Enjoying food is about using all your senses and noticing all the little details. It isn't so much of a stretch to compare food enjoyment to really enjoying sex; you won't until you are no longer frightened and take some time. It also takes buying in to a less-is-more attitude: eating less and enjoying more.

OTHER PEOPLE'S RESTAURANTS

I'm a chef, and it is my job and my passion to eat and drink. I can't wait to try the new restaurant in town just when it opens. I talk about food when I'm not cooking or eating something. I can't get enough of it. The problem is that it catches up with you after a while. I hit 30 a long time ago and the body started to change. As my grandpa used to say, "This getting old is no good." So now I eat smart and it isn't as difficult as I thought. You can still go out to other people's restaurants and eat healthy; it just takes a little extra cross-examination of the waitstaff. Who knows, you might even find a new friend. Remember just because you go out to dinner doesn't mean you have to eat everything on the menu. Eating out is akin to eating at home. It's making the right choices—eating healthy but making sure to have fun, too.

You don't have to eat the whole basket of crusty bread; instead, have one slice or pass on it completely (some breads are "not worth it"). You know it makes you full and really is just empty calories. Save room for the fun stuff that the chef has put his heart into. For me, once I started on bread I couldn't stop. So I "just say no to bread." Don't be afraid to split an appetizer with whomever you're dining, and choose not to order fried foods as a first course. Try to choose light, small appetizers. Appetizers are often the most interesting part of a menu, so why not have two appetizers instead of a main course. Some of my favorite types of appetizers are carpaccios, tartares, and crudos, which are all made of raw or marinated fish. These are wonderfully rich and meaty and make a great light main course. Start with a salad of some type and you are all set. Another option is to split the main course as most restaurants serve huge portions (up to 12 ounces of protein when you really only need 4), so there is plenty to feed two. Remember, restaurants are in the business of making money, and many sit-down restaurants charge a "plate fee" for splitting main courses. This is done not to punish you for sharing, but to cover the hidden costs you may not think of. Manager salaries, electrical and gas charges, breakage, insurance, garbage removal, heating and air-conditioning, and many other costs must still be paid for by food sales.

Finally, most restaurants can do a fruit plate; some are better at it than others, of course. If a pastry chef cares about clients she or he will put something on the carte for those on the MyTendWell Lifestyle Plan or other healthy eating regimes. If you are celebrating, or even if you're just aching to enjoy a sweet, split a dessert. Remember, if you know you are dining out in the evening, take time during the day to think about your meals. Eat lean and save up for your splurge, but don't skip any meals because food keeps your engine running and helps you stay strong willed when the chocolate mousse gets passed around at dinner. Enjoy a couple glasses of red wine; it's full of antioxidants and some believe wine will help stave off great hunger and the temptation to make a complete glutton of yourself.

By consciously making an effort to think about your food choices throughout the day, you can enjoy dinner in other people's restaurants. "Break bread" without eating too much of it. Take advantage of the opportunity for you and your dining partner to try different dishes, talk and laugh, and get a little silly. Sharing food and

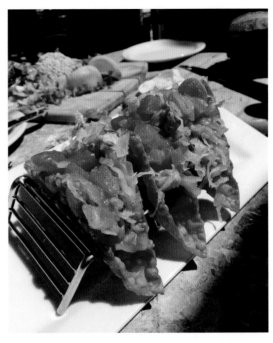

Other people's restaurants, tuna taco.

time together with family and friends in restaurants gives you time to relax and de-stress. You don't have to do the shopping or the dishes either. It is hoped the chef will show you variety and skill, which will keep your palette happy and inspire you to try new healthy recipes at home. Don't forget to keep eating smaller portions of animal proteins, starches, and fats because these are what "get" you. Chefs are masters at hiding the stuff in the most unlikely places.

SHOPPING WITH NEW EYES

Once you have made the commitment to eating healthier, reducing portion size, banishing those starchy carbs, sweets, and snacks, and increasing intake of fruits, vegetables, fiber, lean meats, and fish, you will find you shop differently. You'll spend most of your time in the produce aisles, with a few stops at the fish and meat counters, and barely any stops in the aisles that contain all the unhealthy stuff you previously filled your cart with. You can treat yourself to quick shopping more often. When cooking and

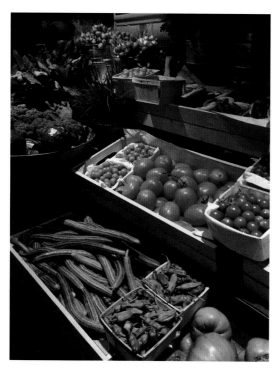

Shopping with new eyes (assorted summer produce, seasonal canned goods, artisanal breads, chilies).

Wild foraged ramps.

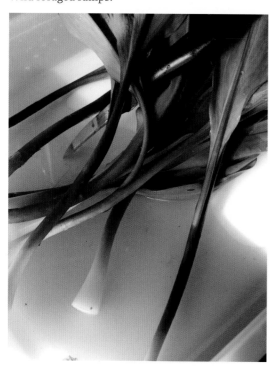

eating are joyous, shopping becomes one of life's pleasures.

Learning to shop with new eyes means taking the time to plan ahead for wholesome, nourishing meals. There's no doubt that you must think about food more than you are accustomed to; some effort must be made to research recipes and to learn how to cook. If you are not skilled at cooking, this is probably the greatest challenge. In the end, however, a great deal of satisfaction can be achieved by taking the time to think about food, read a recipe, write down the ingredients, shop for the ingredients, and produce a meal. When your time is already taxed, it may appear to be an enormous task just to eat, but simple, clean food is quick and easy once you've realized the enjoyment.

Ultimately, however, as you pull away from the convenience of fast food and a poor diet, you will reap the benefits of taking time to shop with new eyes and then eating healthier. It is a fact that nutrition plays a pivotal role in the maintenance of health, the prevention of disease, and the management of chronic conditions. It seems only logical to get out there and embrace what is often thought of as a chore and shop till you drop with *self-love and a healthy pair of new eyes.*

FIVE SMALL MEALS: A DAY IN THE MyTendWell LIFESTYLE PLAN KITCHEN

When a nutritionist friend told me I had to eat more, not less, to lose weight, it was music to my ears. I wasn't ignorant about healthy eating, but I hadn't learned some of the basics that really made sense. For instance it is easy to understand that the body is a machine and you have to give it fuel to run. What is hard to understand is that the less you eat the more your body tries to save in case there is nothing to eat later. The MyTendWell Lifestyle Plan Five Small Meals is a concept that is meant to keep your body energized and working without putting fat away for a rainy day. It is rather like fooling it into believing that there is no need to store fat. So you'll then have the opportunity to burn off some of that spare tire you've been carrying around.

Hard scientific evidence shows that whether you are "eating right for your blood type," fingering through Dr. Weil and Rosie's recipes, calling on Atkins, juicing like the best of them, climbing over the rainbow diet, or sugar busting . . . a few factors remain steadfast. Paying attention to what you eat and exercising regularly may save you from the prevalent, disabling illnesses of the twenty-first century. Poor dietary and lifestyle habits such as inactivity and sedentary behaviors can get you a ticket to many of the following diseases: heart disease, diabetes, osteoporosis, and many cancers. But no matter who is writing the new dietary trend, pretty much the same thing is being said, "If you don't think about changing your dietary habits, you may be in for a long haul of disease and disability."

Eat five small meals a day: three small meals and two snacks. Reduce portion sizes so that you become accustomed to eating a little less, but more frequently. Always start the day with breakfast. It is the most important meal of the day. Try something different every day, such as Irish oatmeal with nuts and a tablespoon of maple syrup. Have a small bowl, not enough to papier-mâché a building. Avoid eating those little packages of microwavable cinnamon raisin instant oatmeal; they are highly processed and contain a great deal of sugar. Try two eggs with a little real cheese (not processed) and one piece of whole-grain rye toast, or two eggs in a whole wheat tortilla with a little salsa. Eating a three-egg omelet with potatoes, two pieces of white bread toast, bacon, sausage, and bad coffee is definitely not a balanced breakfast. First off, it's just too much food, and second, it's just bad. Believe me, I've spent a Sunday or two on the couch vegging out after that kind of mistake. It zaps you of your energy and leaves you feeling hung over even if you didn't overdo it the night before. Simply adjust your favorite breakfast by making an egg-white omelet, putting organic, whole-grain wheat products in your toaster, and

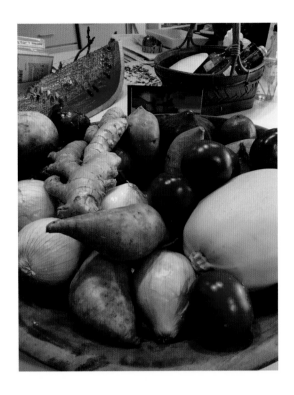

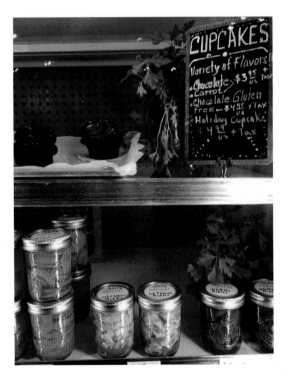

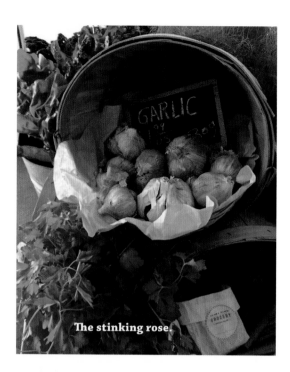

The stinking rose.

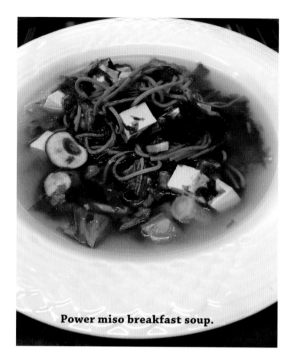

Power miso breakfast soup.

adding a bit of fruit when you're looking for fast and lasting energy in the morning.

Read the labels! If sugar is the first ingredient in cereal then don't buy it. There are plenty of healthy cereals that don't taste like cardboard and don't have incredible amounts of sugar in them. Five grams of sugar per serving is enough. Cereal should have at least 6–8 grams of fiber per serving. This will help reduce the hunger you feel from eating starchy, sugary cereal. A smoothie with protein powder and berries is another good start to the day, and certainly better than a white bagel smothered in cream cheese, or a bowl of Sugar Pops with white toast and grape jelly. Consider trying something from a totally different culture like my power miso soup. The Japanese start almost every day with a similar meal.

Balance animal and vegetable protein. Chicken, fish, and lean meats are good sources of animal protein, and legumes combined with brown rice are a good source of vegetable protein. Cut out the starchy carbohydrates: white pasta, bread and rice, pretzels, cookies, white flour crackers, and anything with hydrogenated oils. Replace those with an abundance of fruit (apples, pears, plums, berries, figs, pineapple), dark green leafy vegetables (kale and collards), orange vegetables (such as squashes and yams), different lettuces, artichokes, asparagus, fresh peas, spinach, leeks, and baby turnips, just to name a few. Pasta is not "Satan's creation," but it isn't something you should eat as a main course 4–5 times a week, especially if you are a carb addict or are overweight. Believe me I've been there, and, like any habit, it is hard to break. You will fall off the organic wagon, but you always have the next day to get back on. Try whole-grain, bean, or rice pastas if you really need a noodle "fix." Once you've found your proper weight, you can make deals with yourself: meatball grinder = 45 minutes running. It actually becomes a fun challenge and a great way to show yourself some self-respect.

It's not about how many times you fall, but how many times you get back up.

Have two small snacks to get you through until it is time for the bigger meals (what could be better than that?)—Finn Crisp crackers with a small piece of cheese or a little natural peanut butter (no hydrogenated oils or added sugar in that peanut butter), or a handful of whole roasted, unsalted almonds. Snacking on healthy food will help stave off cravings for bad sugar and carbohydrate snacks. But no matter what you are eating, the portions should be small: protein no bigger than the size of a deck of cards and a big handful of vegetables. And, there should be variety. By eating balanced portions five times a day, without all the starchy carbohydrates, you will feel fuller and less inclined to eat the candy, potato chips, donuts, cookies, cake, and soda. If you have one starchy carbohydrate for breakfast such as a piece of whole-grain toast, then you don't have a sandwich for lunch. Once a day . . . that's it. Pasta, potatoes, and rice should be a treat for the person who is a carbohydrate addict and trying to lose weight. Some people can eat anything they want and never gain weight, but, for overweight people who skip meals, don't exercise, and are feeling fatigued, starchy, refined foods with sugar and additives should be strictly eliminated from the diet until balance is achieved.

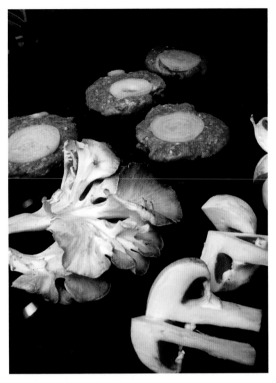

Grass-fed beef burgers with mushrooms.

If 60–65 percent of your diet is plant food, combined with protein and healthy fats, you will begin to look and feel better. The macronutrients, micronutrients, phytonutrients, and fiber will bring wholesome nourishment to the body. Micronutrients are vitamins and minerals. Fiber is the soluble and/or insoluble component of plants that helps move food through the digestive tract. Fiber also has health protective effects by producing short-chain fatty acids that nourish the lining of the colon. Phytonutrients are plant chemicals that have disease-fighting effects and are found in fruits and vegetables. By balancing the protein, carbohydrates, and fats, you'll be more satiated after a meal because the protein takes longer to digest along with the fiber in the vegetables. More fiber and more vegetables, less starchy carbohydrates, and your body won't have extra sugar to store as fat. By reducing starchy carbohydrates and eating more fiber, you can decrease cholesterol and triglycerides in your

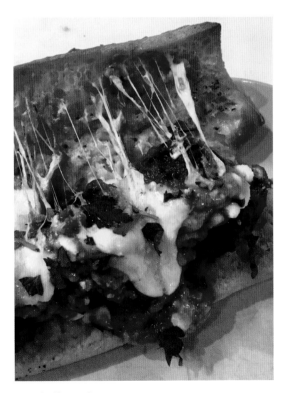

Meatball grinder.

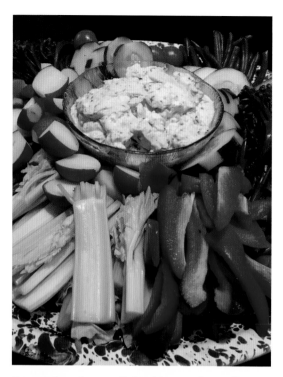

Farmers' market crudités with goat cheese dip.

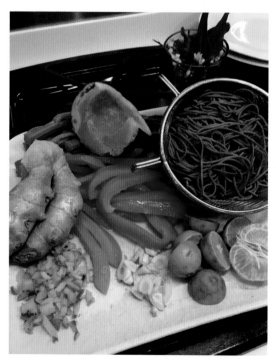

Asian buckwheat noodle sauté.

bloodstream. You need some carbohydrates to get through the day, but the majority should be in a form of plant food other than white potatoes or white rice. Definitely delete all those sweet, high fructose corn syrup drinks. Remember that fruit juice can also spike your sugar levels.

Don't let all these big words scare you. It's really easy. A snack can be as simple as a small apple with a tablespoon of almond butter; lunch, tuna with a salad of watercress, cabbage, radishes, carrots, and sunflower seeds, drizzled with lemon and olive oil and sprinkled with a little salt and pepper. You don't have to be a gourmand to eat well, you just have to be willing to give up your old habits and try new foods. Dinner could be lentils with spinach and garlic. By eating protein with salad or one leafy or cruciferous vegetable, you reduce the amount of calories in a given meal. One day you eat fish with a big, crunchy salad and sautéed spinach. Then the next day, plan a small bowl of black bean soup with chicken sausage and one piece of whole-grain bread. The next, have roasted squash with chicken and an endive salad. Breaking old habits means letting go of old habits. Eating well is not about having starch, vegetable, and protein on a plate. Two vegetables and a small piece of fish or meat actually will come to be more satisfying. Chefs always have lots of great stuff around the restaurant to eat and lots of people to prepare it for them. But even we forget meals and eat the wrong stuff at the wrong time. With proper planning you can shop, then cook 2–3 times a week, and have all your meals covered. If you get your family to help, it can be a fun way to spend the time together. Shopping should be a treat, not a chore. It's all in the way you look at it. Variety is the spice of life, so spend more time in the vegetable aisle.

CREATING NEW TEMPTATIONS

I often feel that I am weak. Why is it so hard for me to say no? Why am I always hungry? Why do I have to have it all instead of being happy with a taste? Why is everything so damn tempting? I've been thinking about this and believe the answer lies in the past. Food has always been important to me, and I often console myself with it during hard times, sad times, stressful times as well as celebratory times. I'm tempted because it makes me feel taken care of, satisfied, and free to indulge in something I find pleasurable. Good food is sensually pleasurable. We like to appease our senses, and, succumbing to temptation, we allow ourselves to indulge in these quiet, sensual experiences. But like the devil in disguise, food can tempt us to disregard what may be better for our health. Result: a sinful mockery of what food should be. Balance. The goal is finding a balance of seductive experiences for all of our senses, a balance that provides a physically nourishing diet.

You can still have a pleasurable eating experience without those French fries we all love, that midnight pint of ice cream after a busy dinner service, or that double cheeseburger on the weekend. As a chef I don't have to eat a whole portion of foie gras terrine or crème brûlée to know if it is perfectly prepared. A tiny taste is truly all I need, more than that my body doesn't need . . . and I really don't have an excuse. Not respecting oneself enough to care about what goes in the mouth is something that will take self-examination. And this can be painful. The best way to start this is to think back and reflect where your yo-yoing stops and starts, and you may be surprised to see a pattern emerge. I know I have found this true. Choosing junk food or overeating good quality food is basically the same thing. Lapses giving in to temptations are triggered in many ways. For some it may be a reaction to disappointing news, depression, or fear, but for others, it may be as simple as a lack of cooking experience, influence of television ads, or just general lack of knowledge about good food, good eating habits, and food recommendations/guidelines.

Many people think eating healthy means eating like a bird or a rabbit, but that couldn't be farther from the truth. Just think how beautiful a produce aisle is with its rainbow of colors. From orange squashes to green and red cabbage, to yellow peppers, purple tipped artichokes, bright green Granny Smith apples, berries of all colors, black and maroon eggplant, red and golden beets, rusty brown mushrooms, dark green poblano peppers, white cauliflower, crispy green kale, speckled yellow bananas, garnet-skinned yams. Even dried legumes, fruits, and nuts are inspiring. Black beans, red lentils, lima beans, black-eyed peas, Brazil nuts, ruby red olives, and hundreds of other tasty and healthy foods are part of a healthy diet and taste much better than lots of the stuff we allow to seduce us. To nature's gifts of delicious fresh fruits, vegetables, nuts, lean meat, and fish, add a little love in the cooking and serving, and you not only have something tempting but something very sexy indeed.

MAKE IT FAMILY STYLE

Growing up, my Grandma had Sunday Dinner every week. We all helped and learned to cook and clean up after. As family moves away and your meals become a table for one, plan weekly dinners/meals with friends. Make at least one weekend meal a family affair in which everyone participates—cooking, cleaning, shopping, whatever it takes—give it a team effort. It is positive time spent with those who are important to you. Time marches on, steal some for good times with loved ones.

Dr. K Tip: Take a 30-minute walk or hike after your dinner, around the neighborhood or at a favorite park or trail. Maybe have a game of watermelon "football." Stretch your legs and burn some energy. But, mostly, spend the time enjoying your company and surroundings.

A DAY ON THE MyTendWell MEAL PLAN

Get up and drink 16 ounces of water.

Break the fast with plain coffee or tea and one of these:

- A smoothie that includes flax or chia seeds, fruit, nut or seed butter, or other protein like dairy, soy hemp, etc.

- Fruit, yogurt, and whole-grain cereal

- Hot cereal, fruit, and nuts

- "Traditional" eggs, veggies, and a healthy starch such as sweet potato or brown rice (great on the weekends when you have more time)

Midmorning—small portion:

- Dried fruit and nuts

- String cheese and dried fruit

- Cottage cheese, berries, and seeds

Water

Lunchtime:

- Greens and protein—raw or cooked greens with eggs, fish, soy, beans, or meat

- Whole grains, a little protein, and veggies—hot or cold quinoa, barley, wholegrain pasta, etc., with all the veggies you want and a garnish of cheese, fish, soy, beans, or meat

- A nice balance of vegetarian starch and protein-beans, corn, and brown rice enjoyed hot or cold as a classic vegetarian salad

- Sandwich or wrap—whole-grain bread or wrap (sprouted-grain products are great), protein like hummus, fish, soy, or lean meat, and all the veggies, greens, and healthy condiments you want

Water

Afternoon crash cancelers—keep these in your desk drawer at work:

- A few nuts or pieces of dried fruit

- Fresh fruit like apples and pears

- Nut or seed butter on veggies like celery or fennel

- Air-popped popcorn with Japanese sesame sprinkles

Water

Dinner—the idea is to use the animal proteins as the side to healthy veggies and starches:

- Roasted, grilled, poached, or sautéed protein—animal or vegetable and two sides (whole grains and a green or fresh vegetable); for example, grilled tuna with quinoa and chard.

- Starchy grain and veggie—for example, barley risotto with summer veggies

- Veggies with protein—Chickpea and Chicken Chili with Brown Rice

Water

Additional snack ideas:

- Water-filled fruits—melons, grapes, etc., frozen or not. I love frozen fruit like grapes.

- A couple of squares of dark chocolate (70% or higher)

Drink more water!

Each day includes 30 minutes of movement. This can be added up throughout the day or finished all at once. Regardless, daily movement is essential to keeping your muscles, ligaments, and tendons strong and flexible.

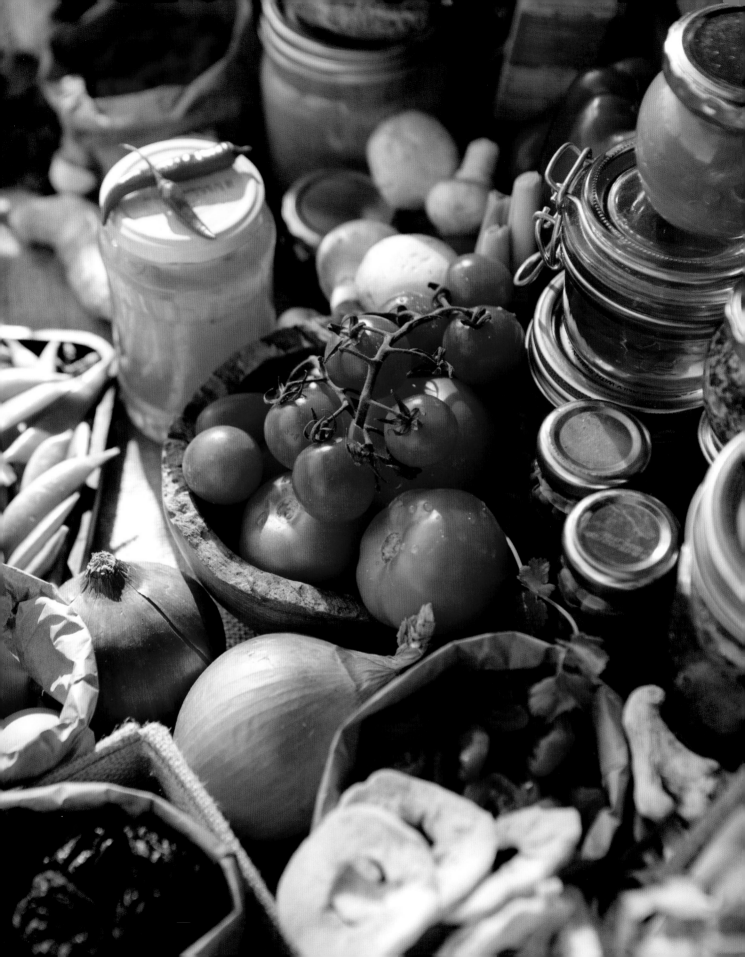

Dipping into the MyTendWell Well of Knowledge

THE MyTendWell PANTRY

A pantry means different things to different people. To me, hearing the word floods me with images of BBC's *Masterpiece Theater*'s century-old tales in the great houses where butlers and cooks scurry around from pantry to drawing room with silver trays full of tea and crumpets. That is a pantry I may have to live without; tea is okay (especially if it is green tea with all its antioxidants) but the crumpets with jam and jelly aren't regulars in a modern healthy eating regime!

Nowadays a pantry is usually a closet crammed full with spices, sugar, white flour, condiments, canned goods, oils, cookies, cakes, crackers, chips, soda, candy bars, cereal, tea, coffee, and convenience foods handy for whipping up a quick meal at a moment's notice. This idea will become as antiquated as the idea of a butler's pantry once you begin your healthy new lifestyle. A healthy pantry is one that should contain little canned food, very little snack food, some spices (no older than six months), some dried food such as legumes, a little whole-grain pasta, some good teas, raw honey, and a few other necessities. A pantry that contains more than 10 percent processed, canned, or packaged food is an unhealthy pantry.

It really makes sense when you think about it—food just should not sit around for too long.

Most food we eat should be fresh and bought within a day or two of serving. The longer food sits around, the fewer nutrients and enzymes are available to provide what we need for our health. And why do we eat food, anyway? First, we eat food for nutrition, and, second, for taste or desire (or is it the other way around? I am a chef after all). Stocking the pantry with soda, junk food, canned stuff, snacks, white flour pasta, white sugar, sweetened cereals, and overly processed convenience foods doesn't leave room on the shelves for the makings of tasty building-block dishes that protect and rev up your wonderful body machine.

My pantry at home is like a tour of the world's cuisines. It's labeled with various ethnic sections, such as Latino, Asian, European, and Southwestern. I love to play with these ingredients when I'm cooking healthy food because each dish becomes a refreshing journey, making cooking healthy and eating more fun. A lot of people, including me, find it hard to eat healthfully if it means eating boring plates of bland, uncreative nutrients. I want flavor and excitement! One thing that must be done, though, is using things while they are fresh, continually using them up so your dishes are as nutritious as possible. Your pantry shouldn't become an old friend who follows you around from apartment to apartment. Foods are meant to be consumed and replaced. Furthermore, grains such as rice and flour left to sit on a pantry shelf for longer than six months will most likely have weevils . . . small wormlike pests that you'd most likely want to avoid eating. "Having friends for dinner" takes on a whole new meaning when you eat them. Any grains such as oatmeal, brown rice, and barley should be stored in airtight containers in the freezer. Oils should be kept refrigerated to keep them from becoming rancid. Purchase oils in dark bottles because light passing through clear bottles results in oxidation; storing the bottles by the stove also targets them for deterioration and rancidity. Always sniff oils if you haven't used them in a while. You will be surprised how quickly they "go bad" if stored at room temperature. Good quality, lightly processed olive, sesame, flax seed, and nut oils deteriorate faster than their highly processed brothers and sisters but offer much more and better flavor and nutritional value. Buy them in smaller quantities and refrigerate to ensure freshness.

We live in an unstable world of abundance and that may translate to overstocking food and everything else in case of emergency. This pack rat mentality, however, creates an unhealthy relationship with food that can lead to insalubrious eating practices. Overstocking the pantry with snack foods will promote the idea that it's okay to constantly snack . . . we think, if the food is there, then eat it! Once in the house, food's an investment that shouldn't be wasted. A conscientious effort should be made to plan meals and buy less food overall. Buy more fresh ingredients and fewer prepackaged items. Long shelf lives do not enhance their nutritional value. Long shelf life usually means foods are preserved with chemicals or have hydrogenated oils in them to maintain shelf life. Chemicals and chemically modified oils only add to unwholesome food choices that lead to ill health.

A healthy pantry is one stocked only with necessities, flavor enhancers, and nutrition providers. This pantry is meant to make your life easier and more interesting because it allows

THE MyTendWell LIFESTYLE PLAN KITCHEN TOOLBOX: TOP FIVE KITCHEN TOOLS

A happy pantry is in a happy kitchen that is stocked full of useful and ecosmart utensils, cookware, and appliances. Chef D knows his way around a kitchen and knows how to move like an athlete on the field. His speed at preparing a meal is amazing. He can literally toss together a delicious meal—breakfast, lunch, or dinner—before I could even figure out what to fix.

To be this efficient, Chef D must have just the right items at hand and he has created a list of his top five kitchen tools so you can create your toolbox, too.

Blender: Vitamix or other high-powered and high-quality blender

Knives: The best-quality kitchen knives you can buy

Cookware: All-Clad or other high-quality, heavy-bottomed cookware

Food processor: Makes preparing and preserving large batches of food quick and easy

Containers: Glass storage containers with lids for all your prepared foods

you to cook with a wider palate of flavors and aromas. On the other hand it shouldn't be overwhelming, making it impossible to control freshness. If you are eating a balanced, wholesome diet that includes loads of fresh fruit and vegetables, lean meat and fish, legumes, oats, and some brown rice, you won't need to fill up your pantry with processed food. You can shop every couple of days and bring home fresh ingredients to base your meals on and use your pantry for inspiration and variety. You'll end up saving your money and your health by using less cash on those prepackaged foods that are full of calories and chemicals and contain no living enzymes or phytonutrients that are so important in a healthy diet. Remember a healthy pantry is a happy pantry.

THE MyTendWell WELL OF KNOWLEDGE

Knowledge is power, and if there is one thing you need to improve your wellness, it is knowledge. Knowing how to achieve optimal levels of wellness is essential for success; therefore, Chef D and Dr. K created the MyTendWell Well of Knowledge—a resource for wellness information for you. The primary resource in the well of knowledge is this book. It provides information and examples for healthy food choices, essential movement, and clean and green living practices all designed to improve your wellness.

There is so much information on health, nutrition, weight loss, and exercise that it is overwhelming. It's coming at you from all angles and from many people. Who's right? Who's not? It's hard to know, but one thing for sure:

if it's quick and easy, it's not a permanent solution, it's a temporary fix at best. MyTendWell is about creating permanent behavior change that will give you the healthy life skills to carry you through life, living and teaching others a wellness lifestyle.

Food for Thought from the Well of Knowledge

Fats (lipids and oils): Fats are an essential component of our diet. Dietary fat is our source for linoleic and linolenic acids (omega-6 and omega-3, respectively), which are needed for growth as well as healthy skin. Fat, or adipose tissue, is also important in protecting our internal organs. Importantly, fat helps with the absorption, transportation, and storing of fat-soluble vitamins A, D, E, and K. (See table 5.1 for classification of fats.)

Carbohydrates are the primary source of fuel for the muscle contractions we perform. Carbs, previously were classified into two groups, simple and complex. Today, these are referred to as nonstarches and starches (or fibers), respectively. (See table 5.2 for classification of carbohydrates.)

5.1 Classification of Fats

Type of fat	Sources found	At room temperature
Monounsaturated	Canola and olive oil	Liquid
Polyunsaturated	Soybean, safflower, corn, and cottonseed oil	Liquid
Saturated	Animal fat, whole milk, butter, coconut, and palm oil	Solid
Trans	Partially hydrogenated vegetable oils, margarine, and shortening	Semisolid

5.2 Classification of Carbohydrates

Class of carbohydrate	Subclasses	Food sources
Simple (nonstarches or sugars)	Fructose, galactose, glucose, lactose, maltose, and sucrose	Fruits, honey, all sugars
Complex (starches or fibers)	Amylose, amylopectic, cellulose, lignin, pectins	Grains, rice, fruits, and vegetables

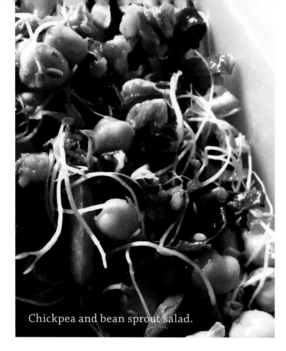
Chickpea and bean sprout salad.

Protein is the primary nutrient we use to build and repair tissue. When wanting to build more muscle we know to increase protein intake. However, it is also important to increase protein in the diet when recovering from an injury, such as after surgery.

Macronutrients are the nutrients we need in grams or larger quantities, such as:

- Carbohydrates
- Proteins
- Fats (lipids)
- Water

Micronutrients are the nutrients we need in milligrams, micrograms, or smaller quantities, such as:

- Vitamins
- Minerals

Dietary Fiber: indigestible forms of starch found in plant-based foods, such as:

- Fruits
- Vegetables
- Grains

Functional Fiber: fiber added to food

Soluble Fiber: fibers that dissolve in water, such as:

- **Citrus**   slows emptying of stomach
- **Oat products**   and glucose absorption

Insoluble Fiber: fibers that do not dissolve in water, such as:

- **Plants (broccoli)** adds bulk to feces and increases
- **Whole grains**   GI motility (movement of feces through intestines)
- **Brown rice**
- **Beans**   may aid in lowering blood pressure

Grains: plant-based foods such as:

Wheat

Freekeh

Barley

Chia

Flaxseed

Quinoa

Brown rice

Wild rice (grass)

Buckwheat

Whole Grains consist of:

- Bran
- Germ
- Endosperm (starchy interior)

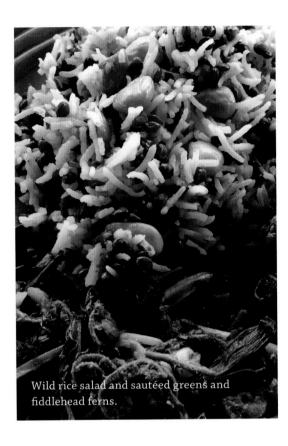
Wild rice salad and sautéed greens and fiddlehead ferns.

ORGANIC FOODS, THE NEW FRONTIER OF AGE-OLD PRACTICES

In the past, organic foods were just a way of life. *Everything* was organic! Back in the good ol' days, there was almost no other way of doing things. Once a less backbreaking way was found, it seemed only natural to head in that direction. Now we've found that the old ways were often the healthiest, and I encourage you to support those businesses that are keeping them alive. It sounds like a noble idea and a dream, but one that I'd love to see come of age in our new century. The food industry and, indeed, the modern consumer desire to find perfection and consistency in a manipulated "nature." Many farmers worldwide have become obsessed with creating new hybrids that look perfect and travel well but miss the boat on flavor and nutritional value. For heaven's sake . . . there are now corn kernels that are part pig! The time for organic is now. The term *organic* simply refers to anything grown or produced without the use of inorganic chemicals. Fruit and vegetables that are called organic are grown without pesticides or genetic engineering in soil that has been free of chemical toxins for a specified amount of time. Organic livestock eat only organically grown feed, and most animals are allowed to roam outside a building. They're not given antibiotics or hormones and generally are treated humanely. Would you really want to eat anything else?

It is easy to label those who support organic farming or agricultural practices as radicals. However, what is becoming more apparent is that organic foods can be more mainstream. People who educate themselves and want quality food not contaminated with toxins will spend the extra shillings to have them. Pesticides have been shown to cause cancer, affect the nervous system, and be passed on to a baby through mother's milk. These are far-reaching consequences that everyone must realize. It IS okay to eat an apple with a few spots that has been grown by a local farmer who respects the land in which he grows food for the public. It's NOT okay to eat perfect-appearing food sprayed with organochlorines such as DDT or chlorophenoxy herbicides such as 2,4,5-T (which is Agent Orange) to satisfy the chemical lobbies in Washington. That's just cray cray . . .

Pay close attention to this: in some places in the United States, produce is actually being irradiated with gamma rays to kill all the organisms and make the products last longer for shipping and for shelf life. Most of the USDA laws indicate that only wholesale packaging must state this fact so the smaller portions we buy in the grocery store possibly do not indicate that we are purchasing, cooking, and eating meats, fruits, vegetables, and spices that have been treated with radiation. Fruits and vegetables are supposed to have helpful living organic components in them; with radiated foods we are actually eating dead food. Scary! Items that are grown locally or that are marked organic definitely become desirable, right?

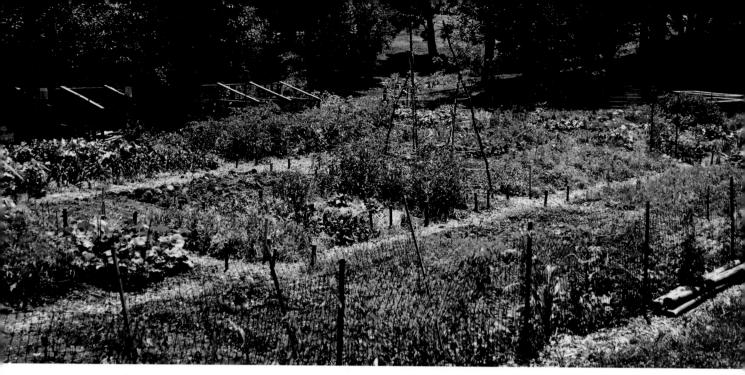

Bloomington Community Garden.

Many people believe that agriculture is dependent on pesticides and herbicides. However, as more people learn that food doesn't have to look perfect to taste good and be good, the sooner we start saving the environment from the toxic residues left over by agroindustrial pollutants. Luckily some supermarkets are selling locally raised fruits and vegetables. That helps maintain relationships with local farmers in order to support their efforts. Farmers' markets deserve support. I'd love to see more and more local chefs creating menus featuring the local organic foods, setting the example for their guests, and showing the availability of good quality, fresh, local produce. We are all responsible for supporting organic, locally grown or raised foods. I even grew organic herbs on my rooftop to use in cooking at my New York City restaurants. I did the same while living in Anguilla at the gardens at CuisinArt and even at home up on Old Ta (the highest point on Anguilla). Food doesn't need to be prepackaged, genetically engineered, picked out of season thousands of miles away and sprayed with wax. Good food can be organic, unpolluted, and harvested, if not right at home, at least nearby.

Now that I'm living back in the Hoosier State I have much more opportunity to use locally grown, homegrown, and organic foods. I forage wild herbs and mushrooms in the woods around my cabin, grow herbs, vegetables, and fruit at my mother's home, and work with the farmers on our farm, Kolb Homestead, to produce foods for the restaurant and for my home kitchen. It is also wonderful to work with a wide range of farmers in the Bloomington area who grow produce and raise animals that are happy and healthy both at the farm and then on the plate.

TOFU, THE SCARY WHITE STUFF

So plain, so bland, so misunderstood! Tofu is the ugly stepsister in the world of protein, but, as is often the case, when she is dressed up and perfumed, her porcelain jiggle can be transformed into something absolutely breathtaking. Tofu is made of soybeans. Soybeans are small legumes or beans that are an excellent source of vegetable protein and calcium. They are also something that grew in endless fields that surrounded my Indiana boyhood home. We never thought of them as food—who'da thunk that soy is one of the most important food sources in the world. Soybeans are used to make soy sauce and tofu (bean curd), soymilk, and soy yogurt. Fresh, they are called edamame, a popular snack food in sushi restaurants. Tofu is a useful food source for vegetarians; soymilk and yogurt are healthy alternatives for people who have intolerance to dairy products. Tofu is made by soaking the ground beans and then adding water to make a puree that is then strained and boiled to produce curd, almost like a cheese. The curd is formed, drained, and then packaged for market. Soy has been a major food source in China for thousands of years. Regular intake of soy has been proven to have many health-protective effects, but even with all its benefits, soy is still maligned. Americans find it one of the scariest of all foods. Just mention the word around any all-American male and he will pale in fear.

With such good news why are we so frightened? Even my friend Christopher, who is Filipino and whose mother tried to raise him on the stuff, squirms at the mention of tofu. It must be the texture. My staff at FARMbloomington seem to have gotten on board, but it has taken many "staff meals" of tofu to get them there. Americans aren't used to the custard thing: it's okay as a dessert flan or the trendy panna cotta but not as our protein! Not for Sunday dinner! We want something we need a knife and a fork for. We want meat! Just remember there are now many ways to work tofu into your diet and once

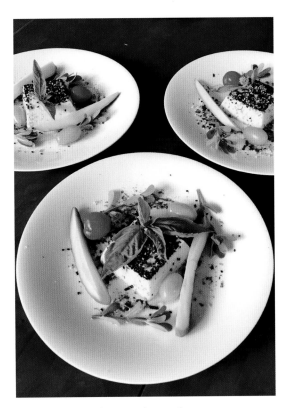

Tofu custard with cucumber and sesame.

you become used to it you'll never give it up. It can truly be something wonderful. Remember our mantra, "Balance."

The benefits of soy are extensive. Soybeans are rich in the isoflavones genistein and daidzein, phytonutrients that have been shown to have protective effects against breast and prostate cancer. It is also a wonder food for middle-aged women going through menopause because it contains a high amount of plant estrogens. Disease-fighting substances called *lignans*, which are found in soybeans, can fight viruses, bacteria, and fungal infections. In addition, soybeans are rich in potassium and have been shown to relieve high blood pressure. Several studies have revealed that soy protein eaten daily can decrease LDL cholesterol (low-density lipoprotein or bad cholesterol). It has also been suggested that the isoflavone daidzein in soy may help decrease the leaching of calcium from bone and therefore reduce the risk of

ALTERNATIVE AND LEAN PROTEIN OPTIONS

Finding alternative and lean options (not "facts") for protein is important. Cooked red meat may be linked to the development of breast cancer, whereas protein sources such as poultry, fish, eggs, legumes, and nuts are not. Try a little tofu, all organic if possible.

osteoporosis. Although not fat free, it is low in fat and high in protein, which makes it the perfect food for weightlifters. So, People, get over your fears and make room at your table for some tofu!

Through the years I've come up with ways to incorporate tofu in dishes by making it more Western. By turning it into a healthy dip, a cream cheese replacement, or a sandwich spread, it no longer seems so foreign. Try diced firm tofu in a Caesar salad made with a tofu Caesar dressing or BBQ'd tofu in a pita pocket sandwich. The uses will soon become endless. I have also developed recipes that use its custard-like texture to advantage. I've created tofu "crème" brûlée that is guilt free. Once you've welcomed tofu with open arms you can venture into ethnic markets and restaurants to see how it is used in the other cuisines of the world and take that knowledge back to your kitchen to experiment.

Tofu may seem bland or boring to many meat eaters out there, yet it is a healthy alternative to animal protein sources. With a little imagination it can be a tasty, healthy food for you and your family. Don't forget one of the most important reasons that tofu should be in your

"AT-A-GLANCE" GUIDE TO TOFU

Silken: Try in sauces, vinaigrettes, dips, creams, and as custard cubes in Asian broths

Firm: Make "cream cheese" and use as a thickener in dips and spreads

Extra Firm: Use in dishes in which tofu is the center of attention. Firm tofu stands proud.

Smoked, Barbecued, and Herbed: Found in some high-end gourmet and health food stores. These are usually flavored extra-firm varieties and are great in sautés, pastas, stir-fries, and tossed salads.

Fresh vs. Packaged: I used to buy fresh tofu from tubs of water in Chinatown or even at my Asian deli when I lived in Manhattan, but when using that, I always cook it. Use pasteurized packaged tofu for uncooked sauces and creams. There is a family that makes homemade tofu in Bloomington and it is awesome. Try a local producer if you have one near you. It is worth the effort. Or experiment and try making it yourself. It isn't that difficult . . . if you know how!

Note: Most firm or extra-firm tofu is better when some of the liquid is removed. To do this, turn a plate over on a small tray to catch the liquid. Place the tofu on the upturned plate and weight it with a second plate; let the tofu sit for 15–20 minutes then drain, and continue with your recipe.

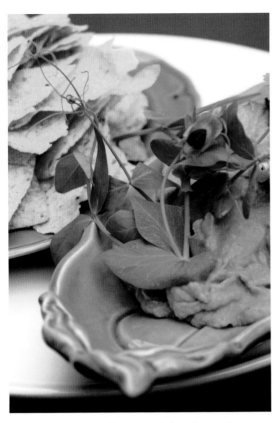

Tofu and green pea "guacamole" with tortilla chips.

pantry—economics. Tofu is pound for pound the best deal when in the market for a health protein to cook with. Tofu is like an edible sponge, absorbing whatever your mix with it creating a truly tasty treat from this often misunderstood food.

RAW FOODS, JUST THE FACTS

Over 60 years ago, Dr. Edward Howell in his book, *Enzyme Nutrition* introduced the importance of food enzymes in human nutrition. He recognized that what may be lacking in the human diet may make us susceptible to many of the degenerative diseases we are afflicted with today. He states that eating food in its natural state unprocessed and unrefined is vital to good health. Enzymes are the substances that are responsible for every chemical reaction that occurs in the human body. Without enzymes, no mineral, vitamin, or

hormone can function. Metabolic enzymes power all of our organs, tissues, and cells; therefore, proper digestion is required for optimal health.

Our bodies naturally produce powerful digestive enzymes in the mouth, stomach, liver, and pancreas that help break down food into smaller particles for digestion in the small intestine preparing for entrance into the bloodstream. Since most raw foods contain their own enzymes, they nutritionally assist in the digestion of foods before our own enzymes are required to break them down. This beneficial concept is especially important because, as we age, the supply of our digestive enzymes begins to wane. Using less of our own enzymes and more found naturally in uncooked foods, such as fresh fruits or vegetables, or those found in predigested foods, such as fermented or aged foods, will help keep us from depleting vital enzyme resources.

If our digestive capacity weakens, acute and even chronic health complaints can occur. Consuming solely processed and cooked food on a continual basis will exhaust our digestive enzymes. Those "worker bee" enzymes, which are trying to keep large particles of undigested food from ending up in the gut, are vital for a happy body. Since food particles need to be minute for entrance into intestinal cells, it only makes sense that large food particles will disrupt the health of the digestive tract. Digestive dysfunction can lead to nutritional deficiencies, dysbiosis

Beet and chard greens in the garden.

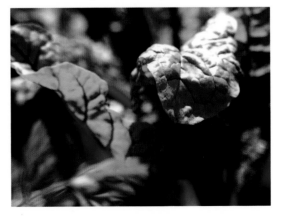

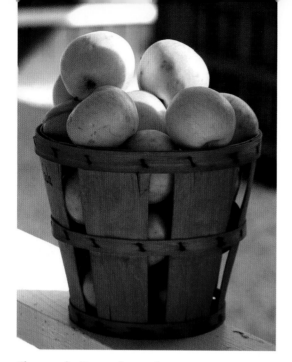

Chesapeake Bay apple stand.

(toxic bacteria infesting your intestinal tract) and many other common problems such as gluten intolerance from grain products, leading to irritable bowel syndrome and celiac disease. Digestion is compromised by improper eating, hormones, psychological state, and lifestyle habits.

Remember, eating a (raw) apple a day may actually keep the doctor away.

A SEA VEGETABLE A DAY KEEPS THE DOCTOR AWAY

Evidence from Stone Age burial sites has shown that seaweeds have been part of the human diet for thousands of years. Not only are sea vegetables low in fat and high in potassium, iodine, calcium, magnesium, iron, and fiber but seaweeds also offer a host of other health benefits.

Traditionally in the East, certain types of seaweeds have been shown to play a role in weight loss by improving water metabolism and by cleaning up the lymphatic system, as well as by helping to alkalize the blood. They have been shown to help the thyroid gland function properly and to offer anticoagulant effects. Seaweeds appear to relieve hormonal imbalances and can be used to treat goiter, high blood

pressure, prostrate problems, skin diseases, and, in Japanese studies, they have been shown to stop mutation of certain cancerous cells.

While I was living in Anguilla, I enjoyed finding out about sea moss and other edible seaweeds gathered there. If you have any other information on local sea vegetables please contact me at kitchdorr@aol.com. I look forward to learning more about the local varieties and local folklore.

Sea vegetables are available in different forms, such as sheets, flakes, granules, and powders. They can be added to soups as thickeners or mixed with sesame seeds and sprinkled on brown rice or fish. Including sea vegetables in the diet is a healthy way to add bulk to meals and, because of their high fiber content, they are filling and thus are a good part of a weight loss plan.

Quick Tip: Many types of sea vegetables exist. Below are a few examples available in Asian markets and over the internet.

Wakame: Deep green, curly leaved. Has been shown to be good for the complexion.

Dulse: Red and blue in color, dulse can be substituted for spinach or eaten like chips once dried and toasted.

Nori: Rich in iron and calcium. Can be bright green to purple in color.

Kombu: Wide and flat, kombu is rich in calcium and helps tenderize legumes.

Irish Moss: Good source of iron. Reddish purple to reddish green in color. Irish moss is used as a source of gelatinous carrageenans, which help to gel food.

Red or White Agar: Used as a food thickener. Red or white agar is available as threads or in powder.

Source: Amanda Ursell. *DK Complete Guide to Healing Foods.* London: Dorling Kindersley Publishing.

WAY TO GO H₂O

When I lived on the Caribbean island of Anguilla, I was surrounded by water but I still walked around thirsty! I know that we can't drink seawater, but with the seven shades of blue that surrounded me 24/7, it should at least have been a reminder to take a sip more often.

Water is the largest single component of the body as it makes up 65–80 percent of total body weight. It is one of the most important and abundant inorganic substances in all living systems. Nutritionally, water helps to break down large nutrient particles during digestion, and, in the gastrointestinal tract, it helps to moisten foods, which aids in their smooth passage. Water has these and many other important functions. Without it, the functioning of organs, including the brain, may be seriously affected. (Source: Tortora and Grabowski. *Principles of Anatomy and Physiology*, 8th ed. New York: HarperCollins College, 1996.)

We've all heard that we should drink eight, 8-ounce glasses of water every day. Most of us don't drink that much, and instead replace this vital water intake with coffee, tea, soft drinks, and alcoholic beverages. Alcohol causes dehydration, and drinking these other liquids does not help replace lost fluid as effectively as water. On average, daily water loss totals 2,500 ml/day, through sweat, for example, or diarrhea due to a GI tract infection. The kidneys excrete about 1,500 ml/day of water, and 600 ml/day of water is lost through the skin (400 ml/day through evaporation and 200 ml/day as sweat), the lungs lose about 300 ml/day exhaled as water vapor, and finally the gastrointestinal tract loses about 100 ml/day in feces. (Tortora and Grabowski, 1996.)

If the main source of body water is ingested through liquids and from moist foods, and if we are neither eating enough fruits and vegetables nor drinking enough water, then how are we replacing this lost water? This translates into constant dehydration that puts the organs and other body systems on overdrive. Without water

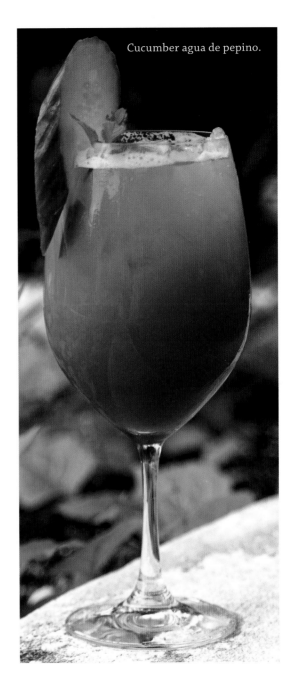

Cucumber agua de pepino.

it's difficult to make enough urine to flush away toxic metabolites and other wastes, maintain proper blood volume, or prevent body salts from getting too concentrated. If you feel thirsty you are already dehydrated. Extreme dehydration can be life threatening. Minor dehydration can make you irritable and tired and make it hard to concentrate. Chronic minor dehydration can

Morning Cleansing Beverage

(Drink on an empty stomach first thing in the morning and follow with plenty of water throughout the day.)

Ingredients:

2 cups purified water

1 tablespoon olive oil

1 organic lemon or lime—washed well and cut into small pieces with peel and pith

Directions:

In a blender combine and blend. Strain and drink each morning for 1 week then once a week afterward to keep your body clean and able.

Note: I like to add a fresh turmeric root, a thumb of ginger, or both for an added kick.

Try using key limes (2–3) or other organic sour citrus.

I often make it for staff or friends with a touch of honey or maple syrup to give it a little sweetness.

IDEAS FOR INCREASING YOUR HYDRATION LEVEL

- Mix water with your fruit juices. A bit of club soda in your juice is like having a homemade soda pop.

- Cut down on caffeine found in colas, coffee, and true teas. These seem like liquids that would be good, but the caffeine actually is dehydrating. Drink herbal teas, both hot and cold. Flavored "spa waters" are easy to make. Just float cucumbers, citrus, or herbs in a pitcher of ice water and allow to sit for 15 or 20 minutes and enjoy any time of the day.

- If going out to a party, drink plenty of water before leaving the house and then a glass between alcoholic drinks. This prevents dehydration and hangovers!

- Drink water to help suppress hunger when starting a new diet.

- Drink before you get thirsty, once you feel thirst you are already becoming dehydrated.

- Always keep liquid consumption up when exercising. It is extremely important if you want to get the most value out of your hard work.

- Eat your water—salads, melons, celery, cucumbers, tomatoes, mushrooms, and many other fruits and veggies are 80 percent or more H_2O. Eat them as snacks or incorporate into meals as often as possible.

- Figure out how much water you should drink (depending on your body size) and measure out enough for the day and take it to work with you. Make sure you finish it before you head home.

- Start the day and end the day with water.

cause constipation; it may also lead to the development of kidney stones and bladder cancer. As we age, we do not recognize dehydration as acutely.

Water has the added bonus of being calorie free. By drinking enough water every day you'll ensure that your body can function at its optimal level. First thing in the morning, before breakfast or a shower, drink a big glass of water. Before a meal, drink water; before you go out to the club, drink water. Don't forget to walk around with a bottle wherever you go. Drink up!

THE HEALTHY PARTY ANIMAL

Going to a party, whether it is for the holidays, a birthday, housewarmings, or just your average Friday night dinner party does not give one liberty to eat everything that is provided by the host. Practicing restraint because you are trying to eat healthy or are on a weight loss plan is perfectly okay. If it's on your plate, you are not required to eat all of it and it is not a reflection on your host's culinary skills. I often offer to bring a soup, salad, or fresh fruit for dessert, that way I know I'm in control of those courses. You can also bring the mixings of a wonderful nonalcoholic cocktail or tart cherry juice instead of wine. Also, try eating a fiber- and water-rich snack, such as veggie sticks and hummus, before you go to a dinner party. This will help keep you away from the cheese and crackers once you get there. At buffets take smaller portions. You can still try a taste of everything, just start by filling 3/4 of your plate with healthier salads and veggies and use the remaining 1/4 of the plate for lean protein and complex carbs.

At a seated meal try asking for a larger portion of vegetables in place of the mac and cheese. It's another great way to enjoy a social get-together without being "that guy" with all the special menu requests. Remember, taking care of yourself is beautiful; what is unappealing is gorging because of an abundance of food or eating for the sake of eating.

Think back to the MyTendWell Lifestyle Plan idea of five small meals a day, this means three meals and two snacks . . . those smaller portions keep calories limited in the body and the surge of insulin low. This is the reason for grazing rather than gorging. A wallet-sized portion of pasta or protein is a serving size. A healthy portion of greens or vegetables is a better alternative to bread slathered with butter. The most important aspect when partying, however, is to make sure you stick with enjoying "a little bit" rather than "a bunch"; that way if you want to have dessert at the end of a nice dinner party, you'll not only have room, you'll feel better on the way home and in the morning.

OUT OF CONTROL

Calories, calories, calories . . .

Studies have shown that restricting calorie intake to 1,500 to 2,000 calories per day is a good way to increase health and longevity. This current research dictates that keeping your weight down, along with increasing exercise, quitting smoking, and drinking less is the way to achieve this healthy lifestyle. The question is, how can we do it?

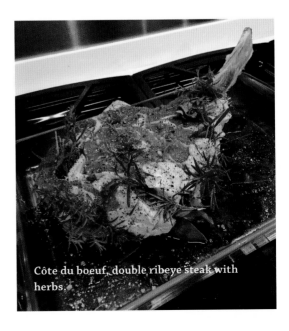

Côte du boeuf, double ribeye steak with herbs.

First of all, there are so many "diets" that it's difficult to decide which one is right for you. All it takes (which may sound trite to most people) is decreasing the portions to half of what you usually eat. I don't know the exact figures for you, but the average American annually consumes 40 pounds of white bread, 32 gallons of soft drinks, 41 pounds of potatoes, and a couple of gallons of vegetable oil to fry the potatoes. That sounds terrible. Per capita consumption of food increased about 8 percent from 1990 to 2000, according to the US Department of Agriculture. That translates to 140 extra pounds of food a year (*New York Times*, July 7, 2002). Fast-food restaurants do supersize portions. Other restaurants serve 20-ounce steaks, which is five times what a portion of meat should be. More than a small fist size, and you've overdone it. That works out to about 3–4 ounces of meat, fish, or poultry. A couple of large portion items, with snacking and high intake of starchy carbohydrates, and you've probably gone way over an average 2,000-calorie a day limit. Beware of those fast-food places moving in to your life!

We are told to clean our plates as we grow up. We're told not to throw away food because it's wasteful. And there's the mentality that encourages bad eating habits, dictating "the larger the better." Feed yourself when you are hungry. You don't need to eat a lot of food to accomplish this. Anorexia is not a pretty picture either, but somewhere between overeating and undereating is a balance that would keep the average person out of the obesity statistics.

Consumption of more fiber helps to decrease hunger, since it takes longer to digest fibrous foods. To eat more fiber you have to eat more fruit, vegetables, and whole grains. This also means if you are eating more of these types of foods you are eating less of the food that can make you hungrier quicker, and maybe less foods that are fried, fast, sweet, and just bad. The healthy food pyramid constructed by Walter Willet encourages vegetables in abundance, and fruit two to three times per day. Nuts and legumes one to three times per day. Whole grains, healthy oils, fish, and poultry comprise a majority of your daily calories. That leaves red meat, butter, white rice, potatoes, flour, pasta, and sweets as a tiny spot that he says to use very "sparingly."

Eating less is actually eating more. Three small meals a day and two snacks can keep you going, especially if you are eating tasty, healthful foods that can satiate even the most diehard fast-food eater. Fewer calories will mean less weight; less weight will mean better health. Eating less calories and less food, doesn't mean you have to compromise on taste. It just means you learn to eat smaller portions of everything ALL the time and be creative and adventurous about new foods.

SO MUCH FOOD, SO LITTLE TIME

Eating processed, fast, frozen, packaged, overcooked, oversalted, denatured (meaning without food enzymes) food, while driving or walking down the street seems to be the way of the world these days, at least on Main Street USA. There is so much beautiful, fresh, organic food available from farmers' markets, supermarkets, and even some innovative food shops and restaurants. It's a wonder why we choose to microwave frozen entrees or eat at fast-food joints. McDonald's drive-through windows are amazing operations. I've seen 20 or more cars lined up ready for empty calories. It reminds me of the farms in the southwest of France. Accept we are like the ducks and geese that line up to be force-fed for future foie gras.

> **Quick Tip:** Foie gras is a dish made of liver from geese and ducks that have been force-fed a high-fat diet. The fowl line up for their corn "gavage" like addicts waiting for the fix.

Sure it takes a little time to think about, and to prepare, WHAT to have for dinner. In reality, however, it takes the same amount of time to microwave or heat up certain frozen entrees as it does to produce a healthy, fresh meal with leftovers that can be eaten for lunch the next day. Most of the dishes in this book are low in animal fats and dairy, and this lack of congealing fat makes them great to eat as leftovers either hot or cold. Talk about efficiency!

It seems that people spend more time researching a new car or computer than they do thinking about what they put in their bodies. Many of the illnesses we experience in the United States are a result of a complete lack of interest in a healthy diet. With so much obesity and chronic illness around, you'd think doctors would spend a little more time counseling their patients on nutrition.

A self-study of nutrition is not a dirty task. What that study effort does, really, is to empower you to take the responsibility for feeding yourself healthy food. That doesn't mean buying Healthy Choice frozen or canned food simply because the label says *Healthy*. Why not research food a little? Take the time to understand food. You don't need a grad school education either. You can go see a nutritionist who will teach you the basics. Go out and buy a cookbook. Take a healthy-cooking class. And, remember, simply being thin doesn't necessarily mean someone is healthy either; a thin body may not be running smoothly and at optimum levels. Eating a wide range of foods, from complex starches (carbohydrates) to lean protein, and good fats along with a rainbow of colors from fruits and vegetables, is truly a way to keep in tune with so much food, so, so little time.

RESOURCES AND WEBSITES

Our Stuff:

MyTendWell.com
www.mytendwell.com

Farmbloomington Restaurant
www.farm-bloomington.com

A Splendid Earth Wellness
www.asplendidearthwellness.com

Additional sites:

Dietary Guidelines 2015-2020
www.health.gov/dietaryguidelines/2015/guidelines

Health Impact News
www.healthimpactnews.com

World Health Organization–Fruit and Vegetable Recommendations
www.who.int/elena/titles/fruit_vegetables_ncds/en/

US Food and Drug Administration
www.fda.gov/Food/default.htm

Mother Earth News
www.motherearthnews.com

Seafood Watch
www.seafoodwatch.org

Eatwild
www.eatwild.com

Civil Eats
www.civileats.com

Wild Edible
www.wildedible.com

Sierra Club
www.sierraclub.org

Ecologist
www.theecologist.org

Rodale Wellness
www.rodalewellness.com

WebMD
www.webmd.com

Centers for Disease Control–Healthy Living–Sleep
www.cdc.gov/features/sleep

Physical Activity Guidelines 2008
www.health.gov/paguidelines/guidelines

Featuring Chef D's Tremendous 20

Take the shopping list that follows to the market with you. If you stick to the items on the list, and only items on the list, you will eat healthfully. You can't go wrong.

Circle items needed from the grocery

- **Water:** Mineral water, club soda, water filters. Stay away from anything with sweeteners.

- **Berries:** Raspberries, strawberries, mulberries, blackberries, blueberries, currants

- **Broccoli:** Heads of broccoli, broccoli sprouts, broccoli florets; also try cauliflower, cabbages, broccoli rabe, asparagus, bok choy.

- **Beans:** Fresh green beans, cranberry beans, snap peas, pea shoots, dried and canned beans, chickpea flour, lentils, black beans, pigeon peas, tiny rice beans; also try prepared bean products like vegetarian chili, hummus, refried beans.

- **Chilies:** Peppers, hot sauce, fresh and dried chilies, salsas

- **Fresh herbs:** Basil, parsley, cilantro, dill, thyme, rosemary, tarragon, sorrel, oregano, and on and on

- **Fruit:** Fresh and dried apricots, raisins, grapes, kiwi, starfruit, papaya, mangoes, pineapple, apples, pears, melons of all varieties, peaches, etc., etc.

- **Garlic:** Only fresh garlic should be used; also try onions, scallions, and shallots.

- **Grains:** Wheat berries, wild rice, brown rice, barley, oats, spelt, frik (Egyptian wheat,) quinoa, teff, amaranth, bulgur, etc. Also, try whole-grain breads, crackers, and cereals. When purchasing prepared whole-grain products, such as crackers, breads, and other baked goods, whole grain must be first on the list of ingredients with little or no processed flour.

- **Tomatoes:** Cherry tomatoes, heirloom tomatoes, also red and orange bell peppers. Also try tomato and vegetable juices, tomato paste, other natural canned and jarred tomato products, and sun-dried and oven-roasted red peppers.

- **Nuts and seeds:** Walnuts, almonds, hazelnuts, and pecans. Fattier nuts like cashews, Brazil nuts, and macadamias can be eaten in moderation. Pine nuts (pignolis), sunflower seeds, and peanuts (subterranean legumes) are often in the same aisle but aren't nuts at all. They are closely related when it comes to nutritional value. Grab some. Stay away from highly salted, flavored, or candied varieties.

- **Lean proteins:** Fresh and frozen turkey, naturally prepared turkey, extra-lean ground turkey; also try chicken, skinless duck breast, wild game birds, bison, ostrich, emu, seafood, and vegetable proteins.

- **Greens:** Spinach, collards, mustard greens, turnip greens, chard, kale, arugula, romaine, mesclun, cabbages, callaloo, etc., etc., etc.

- **Fish:** You'll find omega-3 fatty acids in a wide variety of fresh fish and shellfish in all its many guises. Also try canned, in water, sardines, mackerel, salmon, tuna, and anchovies. Omega-3s may also be found in some natural eggs, wild game, and free-range poultry and livestock. Purslane, a wild weed found throughout the world and some farmer's markets, is one of the plant world's best sources.

- **Soy products:** Firm, soft, and flavored tofus, soy milk, soy cheese, miso, edamame (fresh soybeans). Also try tempeh and other soy products. Read the labels and beware of added sweeteners and chemicals.

- **Spices:** Black peppercorns, coriander, fennel seeds, cinnamon, cloves, star anise, nutmeg, and other dried spices. Also try blended spice combinations like curries, masalas, and Chef Daniel's Kitchen D'Orr Spice Blends at www.farm-bloomington.com.

- **Squash:** Butternut, acorn, pumpkin, sweet dumpling, and other hard "winter" squashes. Also try "summer squash" like zucchini and yellow squash as well as canned pumpkin for an easy soup or vegetable side dish. Also use sweet potatoes.

- **Citrus:** Lemons, limes, grapefruit, oranges, tangerines, etc.

- **Tea:** Green tea, black tea, herbal teas

- **Low-fat dairy:** Plain low-fat yogurt, sugar-free low-fat flavored yogurts, sugar-free low-fat frozen yogurt. Also try other low-fat/no-fat dairy products like skim and 2 percent milk, string cheese, low-fat ricotta, etc.

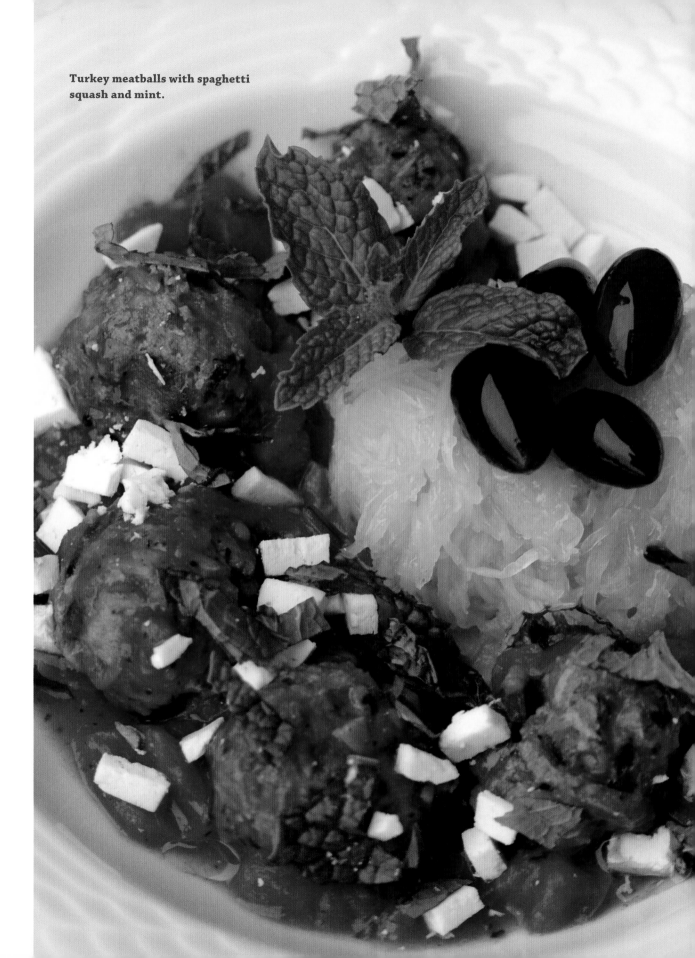

Turkey meatballs with spaghetti squash and mint.

6   The Proof Is in the Pudding

BREAKFASTS

What you choose as that first meal of the day to break the fast from the prior evening's dinner is a very important decision. It may be the most important food thought you will have the whole day! I know it is easiest to do what I used to do, and that was nothing. Just grabbed a cup of coffee, and out the door I went. I'm not sure why many of us want to start the day with dessert, but I think that is probably worse than what I was doing. Doughnuts, sugary "cereals," waffles, muffins, and Cinnabons aren't going to help you shrink your buns, but they are going to start you on the slippery slope of a roller coaster ride of a sugar rush. When I did finally put the effort into a more healthful morning routine, I started feeling better, more energetic, and emotionally stable. To start the new regime, I pulled out my blender and made citrusy cleansing potions and then moved onto smoothies and juices. They were fine, and quick, but I found myself missing chewing, so I created some different egg and grain dishes that get you going on days you have a few extra minutes to spend in the kitchen. In many cases, I have replaced processed foods and starches like potatoes with crunchy vegetables. Yes, I do miss shredded potato hash browns, but I have them on rare occasions and make them with the skins or with sweet potatoes. Now I am switching things up by having a few smoothies a week, a couple grain dishes, and a couple egg recipes and then starting it all over each Monday with a citrusy cleanse. I hope you'll give some of these a go.

Note: All recipes or spice blends referenced but not listed here can be found at **www.farm-bloomington.com**.

107

#1–Chef D's Schwetty Breakfast Butter Balls

Makes 4–6 balls

Ingredients:

¾ cup raw honey

1 cup crunchy organic peanut butter (or other nut or seed butter)

¼ cup ground flaxseed

¼ cup chia seeds

1 cup toasted pumpkin or sunflower seeds

¾ cup shredded, sugar-free coconut

¼ cup dried fruit of your choice, diced, or whole raisins or currants

¼ cup toasted sesame seeds (for rolling)— I like to blend black and white seeds

Directions:

Blend honey, nut butter, seeds, coconut, and dried fruit. Form into 1-inch balls and roll balls in sesame seeds. Put on a cookie sheet and refrigerate for 2 hours or overnight.

Store in the refrigerator, separated by parchment paper in an airtight container, for up to 3 weeks.

#2–Frozen Dark Chocolate Banana "Sushi"

Directions:

Peel bananas and "paint" with melted 70 percent plus chocolate. Roll or sprinkle with nuts, seeds, dried fruit, or granola. Put in freezer. Once frozen hard, put in ziplock bags. Pull from freezer before you get in the shower and enjoy with a cuppa tea before work.

#3—Cha Cha Chia . . . in the Morning—Chia Seed Parfait

You just must add chia to your morning. It has so many benefits that you would be crazy not to. Try this simple, raw recipe for yourself. It is like starting your day with dessert!

Makes 2 healthy servings (or 1 serving each for 2 days)

Ingredients:

4 tablespoons chia seeds

¾ cup low-fat milk or unsweetened nut, seed, or soy milk

2 teaspoons agave, maple syrup, or honey

¼ teaspoons vanilla extract

Pinch of salt

1 cup stone fruit or tropical fruit

½ cup berries

1 cup Greek yogurt (or soy sour cream)

Crunchy sprinkles, such as ground flaxseed, favorite whole-grain cereal, hulled hemp seeds, toasted seeds or nuts.

Directions:

Combine chia, liquid of choice, sweetener of choice, vanilla, and salt. Refrigerate until jellylike (2–3 hours). Stir well and set aside.

Prepare your other fruit by cutting into bite-sized pieces. In a parfait cup or tall skinny glass, begin layering chia mixture, fruit, and yogurt. Cover. Refrigerate overnight or up to 1 week.

Just before enjoying, top with crunchy sprinkles.

Note: This recipe can be doubled or tripled and served in a large-footed glass bowl at a fabulous weekend gathering.

#4—"Wake the Duck Up" Oatmeal

This will either make you feel "just ducky" or give you a morning goose! It is so easy and you can change it up to fit your mood or your pantry. I have a hard time remembering breakfast, but Dr. K says it is the most important meal of the day, and even she has a hard time doing it right. So, do it the night before and you will already know what you are having for breakfast! So "Wake the Duck UP!" to good health.

Makes 2 healthy servings (or 1 serving each for 2 days)

Ingredients:

1 cup banana, chopped

2 tablespoons nut butter of choice

1 tablespoon maple syrup, agave, or
    sugar-free jelly

½ cup quick oats

1 tablespoon ground flaxseed or whole chia

¾ cup low-fat dairy, coconut, soy, hemp, or nut
    milk

1 teaspoon Sweet Season Spices, Chinese five
    spice, or cinnamon

½ teaspoon real vanilla or almond extract

2 tablespoons Greek yogurt

½ cup toasted coconut, tree nuts, seeds, or
    granola

Directions:

In a glass bowl, combine banana, nut butter, and sweetener of choice and microwave 20–30 seconds. Stir well. Add oats, seeds, liquid of choice, spices, and extract, and mix well. Spoon into two serving dishes, cover, and refrigerate overnight. Before serving, top with a spoon of yogurt and sprinkle with crunchy stuff. Enjoy!

#5—Muscle Mud Breakfast Bar

Ingredients:

Makes 8 healthy bars

2 cups hemp protein powder

2 cups hulled hemp seeds

1 cup pitted dates, chopped and packed

½ cup amber raw blue agave

1 cup golden raisins

1 ½ cups water

⅓ cup ground flaxseed

2 tablespoons hemp oil

½ cup cacao powder

2 teaspoons Sweet Seasoning

1 tablespoon freshly ground ginger

1 tablespoon baking powder

Directions:

Combine all ingredients together in a food processor. Line a 12 × 8 dish with parchment paper, spread ingredients into dish, and bake at 350 degrees for 35 minutes. Let cool on a wire rack. Cut into 2 × 3 inch bars. Enjoy!

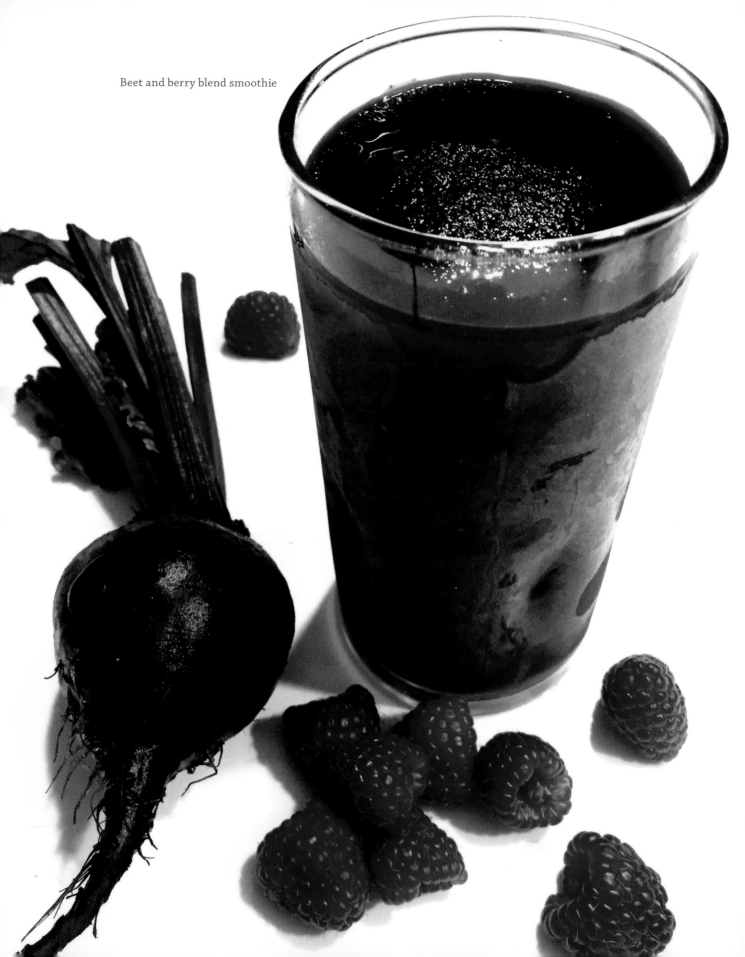

Beet and berry blend smoothie

SMOOTHIES/BLENDER DRINKS

These are a quick and easy way to start the day. They are so versatile that you really don't need a recipe. You can use up practically any raw fruit or veggie you have in the fridge. The key is to get a balance of sweet with the vegetal flavors of hearty greens and other produce. I also love to add a bit of a burn with ginger and the antioxidant powerhouse turmeric.

Please do not only follow recipes! Use what looks best in the market and let the ingredients tell you what to put into your smoothie. These are just some suggestions.

The drinks that follow are created with their colors in mind. We need to think about the colors of our food. Each color usually has different nutritional values. Make sure you use a rainbow of ingredients throughout the day, or all at the same time in your smoothie. Just remember that the more colors you use, the more likely you are going to end up with brown.

Other key ingredients in my smoothies are the chia or flax seeds. They not only add nutrition, but they also bind the smoothie and give it texture. The smoothies are less likely to separate in case you don't drink everything all at once.

I usually make enough to have another glass to put in the freezer. I like to pull them out 30 minutes before dessert time and let them sit at room temperature so they begin to thaw. Then I eat them like one would Italian ice. Or I pull them out just before bed, leave them in the fridge, and have a smoothie waiting for me in the morning.

One major issue is that you need good equipment. I love my Vitamix blender. It pretty much changed my life, like the Cuisinart food processor did in the 1970s. There are now other brands on sale, the NutriBullet gets high marks from a friend, for instance, but I use my blender for a lot more than smoothies. This is one instance when you need to spend more on your equipment.

The Green Hornet

This smoothie has the sting of ginger and the goodness of the greens, making it a perfect eye opener. It will solve the case and keep you safe, just like Kato and the Green Hornet. Mix it up with different seasonal greens and fruits.

Makes 2 healthy servings

Ingredients:

½ thumb ginger

1 medium fresh turmeric root (or 1 tablespoon turmeric powder)

2 large handfuls of greens (kale, chard, beet greens, collards, etc., or a mix)

2 apples, cored and chunked

½ cup fresh pineapple chunks

¼ cup chia seeds

½ tablespoon flaxseed oil

3 cups light-colored liquid (water, coconut water, aloe juice, or combo)

6–8 ice cubes

Directions:

Blend until very smooth, and adjust thickness with additional liquid as needed. Drink it down.

Georgia on My Mind

This peach smoothie is light and refreshing. During peach season, use fresh peaches, of course, and leave the skins on for the extra fiber. Off-season, there are some very good frozen peaches available. I love to eat a handful of blackberries while I'm sipping on this drink. It reminds me of my Georgian friend's peach and blackberry cobbler.

Makes 2 healthy servings

Ingredients:

3–4 large peaches (or 2 cups frozen slices)

2 cups green tea

1 tablespoon agave nectar

½ lime

5–6 ice cubes

Directions:

Combine in a blender and process until smooth. Drink it down.

Kiwi Crush

This is one of my favorite eye openers. People always ask for the recipe, and I'm embarrassed by how easy it is and so tempted to add a few things just to make it sound more technical. Kiwis have a great flavor and are surprisingly a real vitamin powerhouse. They are full of vitamin C, potassium, pectin, and fiber. Most people think of kiwis as a garnish, but here they finally get their place at center stage.

Makes 2 healthy servings

Ingredients:

4 kiwis, peeled

2 cups green tea, brewed

1 tablespoon agave nectar

10–12 ice cubes

Directions:

Blend until smooth. Drink it down.

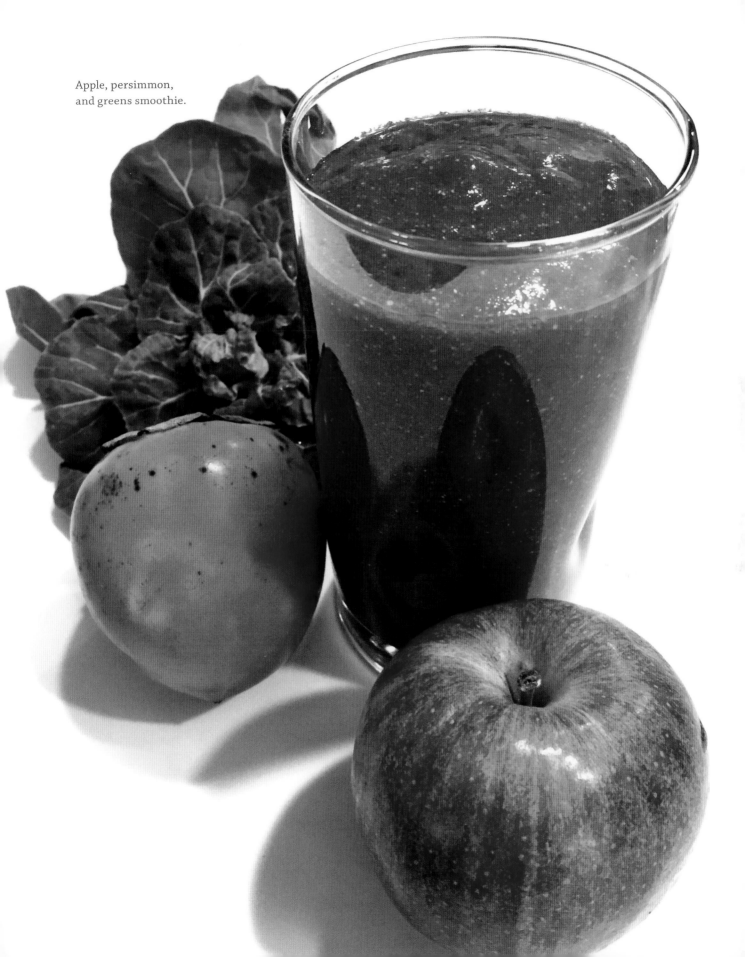

Apple, persimmon, and greens smoothie.

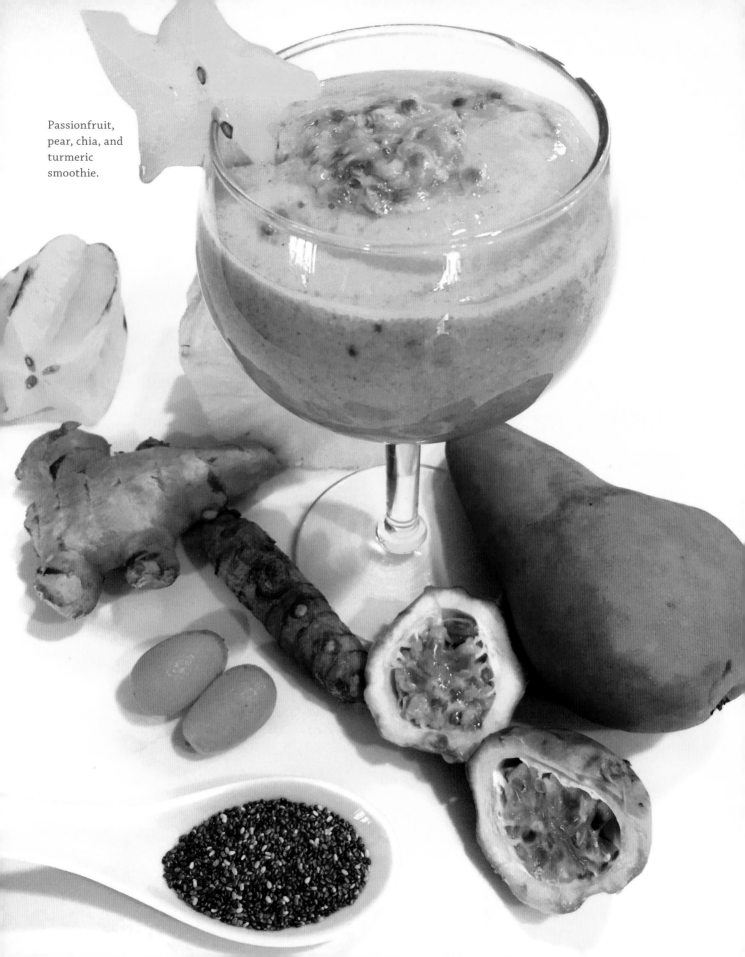

Passionfruit, pear, chia, and turmeric smoothie.

Papaya and Blueberry Breakfast Bomb

This little drink really packs a punch. There are tons of antioxidants in the berries, and the papaya is a great energy powerhouse that will get your day started with a bang.

Makes 2 healthy servings

Ingredients:

½ cup papaya, peeled, diced, and chilled

½ cup blueberries, washed and chilled

1 cup green tea, brewed and chilled

1 tablespoon agave nectar or honey

Juice of 1 lime

Directions:

Place items in a blender and blend until smooth. Drink it down.

Chef's Diet Options:
A bit of soft, custard-style tofu can be added. Frozen berries may be used.

The Cheeky Monkey Smoothie

I like all types of flavors: bitter, sour, vegetal, sulfur, earthy, etc. In fact, I like things that might put a lot of people off—strong flavors of dried shrimp and fish paste, aged game, and funky cheeses. I've even tried to get family, staff, and friends on board with some of my stronger flavor-forward morning potions and smoothies, but not all pass the sniff test with them. Well . . . this is one that does. Everyone is crazy about this nutty, tropical eye-opener, and I think you'll love it, too.

Make 2 healthy servings

Ingredients:

2 tablespoons ginger, minced

1 banana

2 prunes, pitted

2 tablespoons chia seeds

2 tablespoons peanut butter, natural, no sugar added

1 cup yogurt kefir

1 cup water

1 cup frozen fruit (such as mango, pineapple, or peaches)

Directions:

Combine all ingredients in a high-powered blender. Start on low and increase speed to high. Puree until smooth. Thin as needed with additional water. Pour, drink, and enjoy!

KNIFE, FORK, AND SPOON BREAKFASTS

Many folks in the West can't imagine starting their days without bacon and eggs, and I love to as well. There is a time and a place for it, which means not every time or every place. These are some healthy riffs on some classics, as well as some new dishes you may not recognize at all. Remember, change is good, and trying a new recipe that starts the day off in a different way can change your outlook on the rest of the upcoming 24 hours. One thing I've tried to do is cut back on unnecessary fats by developing cooking methods that use the natural moisture in the ingredients, for instance, steaming the eggs gently instead of frying them in vegetable oil. Another method of changing your morning routine is to cut out the processed sugars and white flour and substitute them with interesting grains and sweeteners from around the world. Remember to start the day by eating from a wide colorful palette of vegetables and fruit. You might also enjoy trying some new dishes based on Asian breakfasts that begin the day in a more savory way with miso soup, fish protein, and sea vegetables. When shopping for breakfast cereals, make sure you check the labels and make informed choices. It is almost impossible to find a box of cereal, even in the healthier food section, that doesn't have some sort of sweetener as the second ingredient. It is said that breakfast is the most important meal of the day, and I agree. So if you start the morning right, you are more likely to keep your day going in the right direction.

A note on eggs: I love to begin the day with an egg dish every once in a while. Just remember that the better the egg, the better the dish. In many of the following recipes, I suggest cooking eggs just until the whites are firm and the yolks are runny. When doing this, you don't want to use industrial eggs that have been overprocessed and usually aren't as fresh as local eggs. If you don't know where your eggs are raised, or by whom, you might want to cook them to a firmer texture and higher temperature.

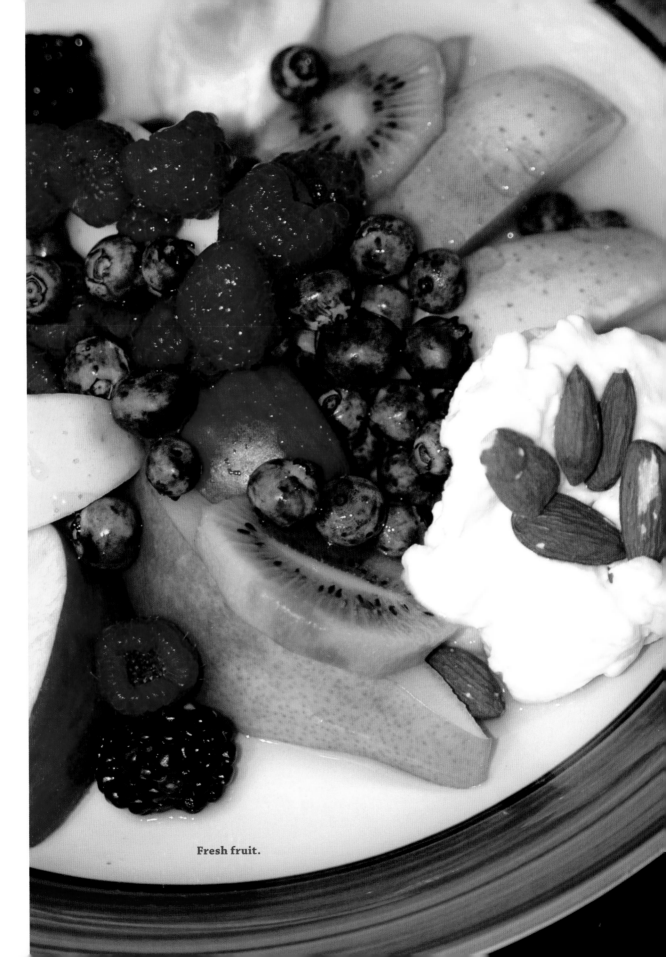

Fresh fruit.

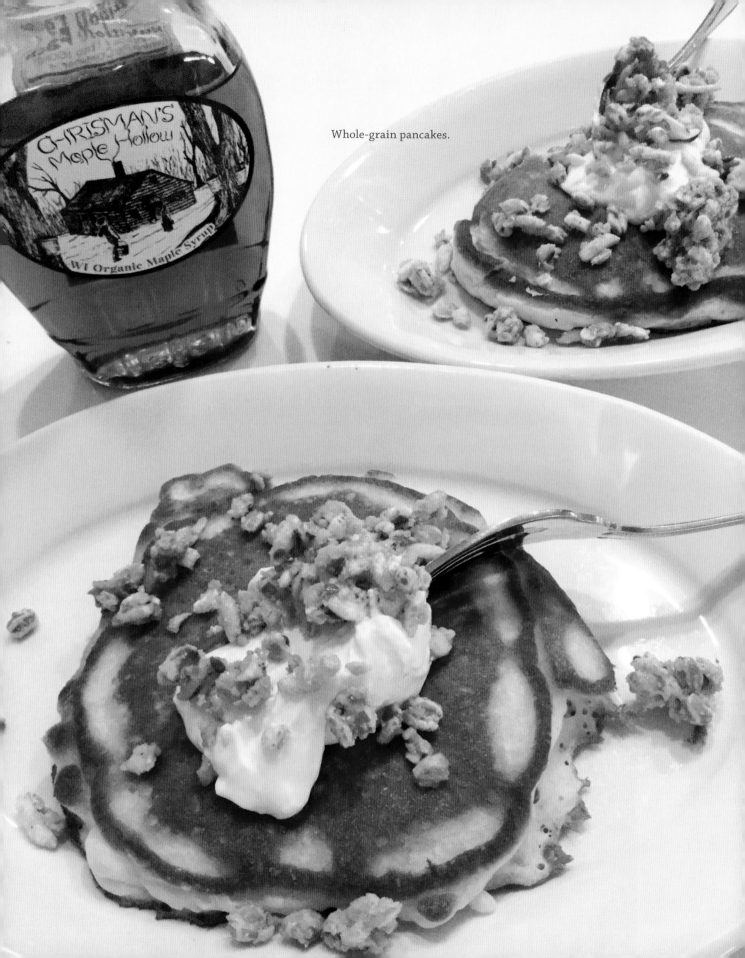

Whole-grain pancakes.

Flaxseed and Agave Pancakes with Yogurt and Granola

These are surprisingly light and airy and will make even the staunchest IHOP disciple a believer in the "fiber fellowship." Top with yogurt and granola, as well as fresh fruit, and you don't even need butter and syrup.

Makes 3–4 healthy servings

Ingredients:

1 cup flour

¼ cup whole wheat flour

¼ cup ground flax seeds

1 tablespoon baking powder

1 pinch kosher salt

2 eggs, whisked

¼ cup olive oil

1 ½ cup low-fat milk

2 tablespoons agave nectar

Granola

Vegetable spray as needed

Optional garnishes: Low-fat yogurt, granola, fresh fruit, berries, agave nectar, and real maple syrup.

Directions:

Combine the dry ingredients and mix well to combine.

Whisk the eggs with the remaining ingredients, and fold them into the dry. Do not overmix or it will toughen the batter. Allow to rest 5–7 minutes. Thin as needed with additional milk.

Cook in a Teflon-coated sauté pan sprayed lightly with vegetable spray. When bubbles form on top, turn and cook until lightly brown on the other side.

Serve immediately with desired toppings.

Baked Eggs with String Cheese, Market Greens, and Cherry Tomatoes

This is an easy way to do eggs because you serve them right in the pan. No flipping or flopping, just good eating. They also stay hot for a while, so if you have late risers you can serve these with whole wheat toast, half an English muffin, or even a multigrain tortilla.

Makes 2 healthy servings

Ingredients:

1 tablespoon olive oil

2 large garlic cloves, minced

2 cups greens (spinach, chard, kale, beet tops, etc.), roughly chopped

10 cherry tomatoes

4 eggs

2 pieces mozzarella sticks or string cheese, finely chopped

Salt and pepper to taste

Directions:

Preheat oven to 450 degrees.

Heat an ovenproof Teflon-coated sauté pan over medium-high heat. Add the olive oil and garlic, and sauté until toasty and golden. Quickly add the greens, and stir to combine. When greens are wilted, add the cherry tomatoes and season to taste with salt and pepper.

Turn off heat and crack eggs over the top of the greens in the pan. Season lightly with salt and pepper. Sprinkle with the chopped cheese, and place in preheated oven. Cook until eggs are set up and yolks are still slightly runny. Serve at once.

Chef's Diet Options:

Use different greens to get different flavors. Choose what is nicest at the market.

Try adding mushrooms or other veggies.

Spice it up by serving salsa on the side.

Try other nonfat or low-fat cheeses on top.

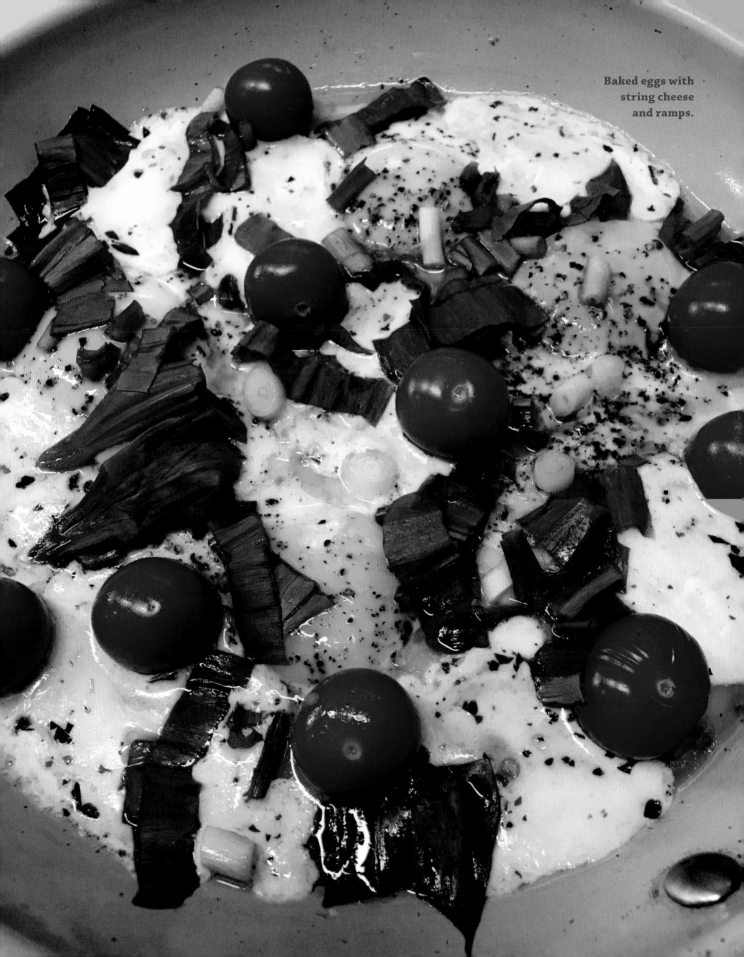

Baked eggs with
string cheese
and ramps.

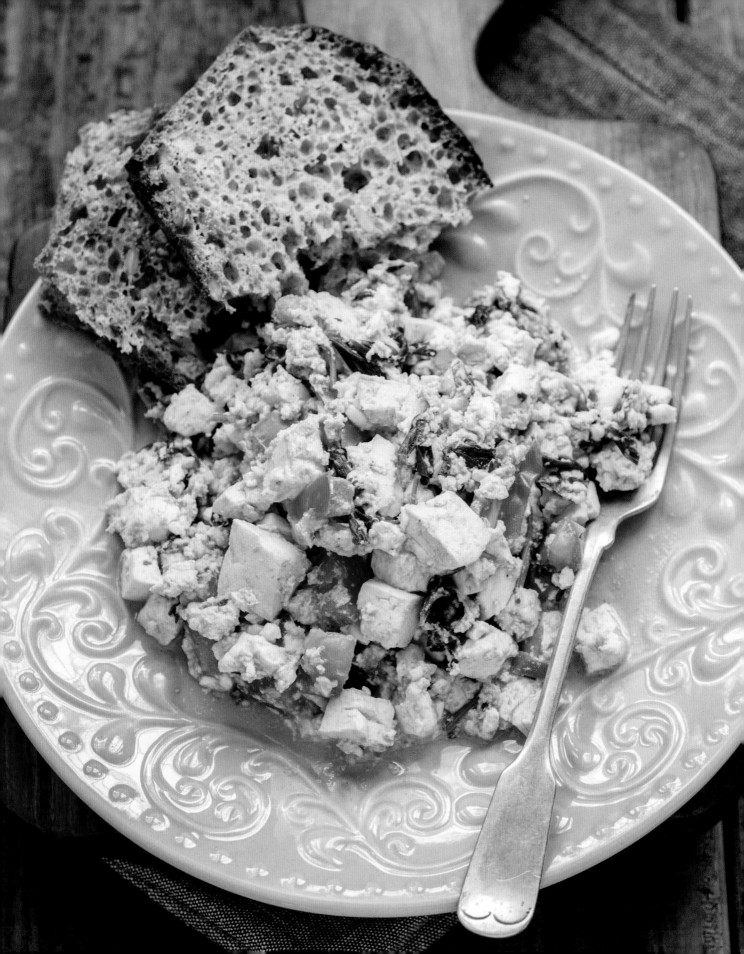

Scrambled Tofu with Garlic and Turmeric

Tofu is a low-fat protein source, and garlic and turmeric are antioxidant powerhouses, so this combination gives you a one-two punch to get you going in the morning. Serve with toasted whole wheat bread.

Makes 3–4 healthy servings

Ingredients:

1 tablespoon olive oil

2 cloves garlic, minced

2 teaspoons turmeric powder

1 pound soft tofu, drained well and lightly crumbled

Salt and pepper to taste

Directions:

Heat the olive oil, add the garlic and turmeric, and cook until tender but not browned.

Add the tofu and stir to coat. Reduce heat and continue to cook for 4–5 minutes until heated through. Taste and adjust seasoning.

Chef's Diet Options:

Add your favorite chopped herbs. I like cilantro, parsley, fennel tops, or basil.

Add veggies. Leftovers or freshly chopped, the veggies add crunch and texture.

Add chilies. They kick up the heat as well as your metabolism.

Add cheese. Traditional, soy, or nut milk cheeses add that great stringy texture. Be sure to add cheeses just before serving, after removing from the heat.

Gardener's Breakfast

This meal will make you feel good. As always, it's all about the ingredients. What could be better than vine-ripe tomatoes, organic eggs, and good ricotta cheese? You can doctor it up with fresh herbs if you like. After this breakfast, you'll feel full, yet light and ready for the day. I call this "gardener's breakfast" because I created it from my mother's garden in Indiana.

Makes 2 healthy servings

Ingredients:

4 eggs

2–4 lettuce leaves (I like arugula or spinach)

½ cup low-fat ricotta cheese

1 large beefsteak tomato, ripe, cored and sliced

1 tablespoon olive oil

½ teaspoon garlic salt

Freshly ground pepper as needed

Directions:

Boil the eggs to desired doneness and peel. Lay down the lettuce leaves on the plate and top with the ricotta, tomato, and boiled eggs.

Drizzle olive oil over everything, and season with garlic salt and freshly ground black pepper.

Chef's Diet Options:

Cook the eggs sunny-side up or poach the eggs.

Add a bit of homemade salsa or pico de gallo for a touch of spice.

Scatter with chopped fresh herbs like basil, parsley, tarragon, chervil, or dill.

Use a mix of heirloom tomatoes.

Add some bean or alfalfa sprouts.

Use nonfat cottage cheese in place of the ricotta.

Quick Breakfast Miso Soup

My friend Mihoko made me this soup for breakfast the first time I visited her in Atlanta, and I fell in love with it. Mihoko made hers from scratch, and I remember her chopping and grating away in the kitchen. I like to figure out quick ways to do things, and the instant miso soups I found did just that. You can purchase good-quality dehydrated soup mixes in the Asian aisle of most supermarkets and just "jazz it up" at home for a quick and satisfying start of the day.

Makes 1 healthy serving

Ingredients:

1 ½ cup water

1 package miso soup mix (plain or with garnish)

¼ pound tofu, diced—I like the custardy soft tofu but any variety will work

1 scallion, cut thinly on a bias

2 button mushrooms, thinly sliced

1 tablespoon dried seaweed, such as hijiki

1 pinch toasted sesame seeds

Directions:

Boil water in a small saucepan and add remaining ingredients. Return to a boil and remove from heat. Taste and adjust seasoning as needed.

Chef's Diet Options:
Add diced leftover poultry or lean meat.
Add chili peppers, sesame oil, and soy sauce to spice it up.
Soak dried mushrooms to add meatiness (shiitake, porcini, cloud ear, or black trumpet).
Poach an egg in the broth as it simmers. I like to leave the yolk nice and runny.

THE MISO MINUTE

Miso is a thick paste traditionally made from fermented soybeans. If you've been to a Japanese restaurant, you've probably had miso in a broth or marinade. There are many varieties of miso made with different additional grains, such as rice, barley, wheat, and others. The most widely used are smooth white and red miso, but there are many other varieties that come in different colors, flavors, and textures. Miso has natural living enzymes that are beneficial to digestion. Most instant miso soups are made with white miso, giving it a light flavor and amber color.

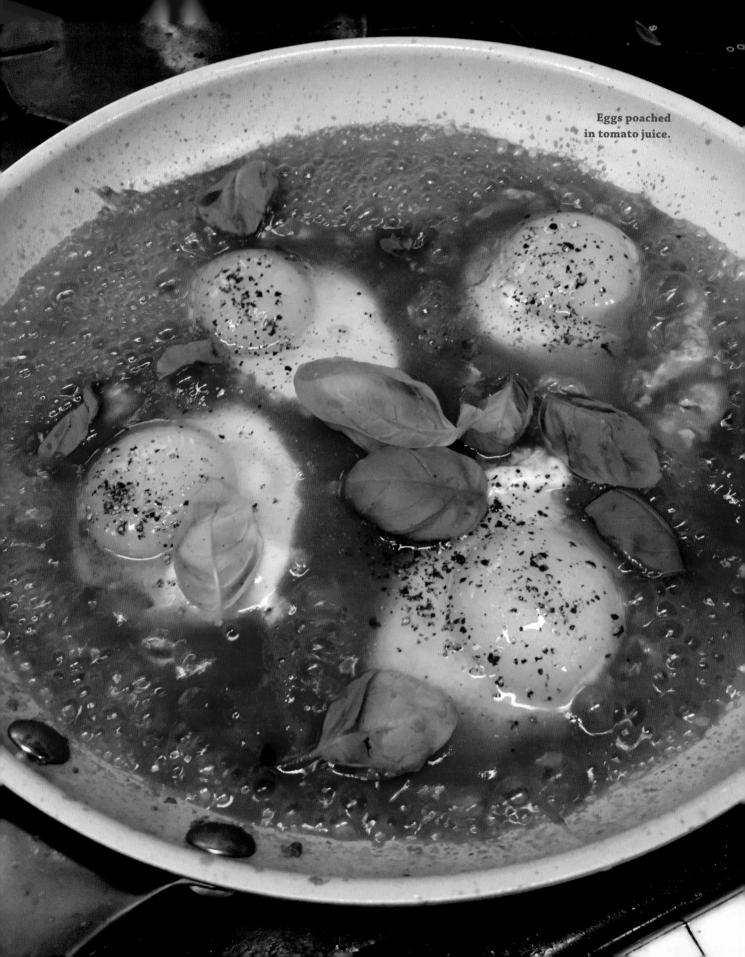

Eggs poached
in tomato juice.

Eggs Poached in Spicy Tomato Juice with Basil and Spinach

This dish is easy to cook for one but can be easily multiplied and done for a crowd. I like to use Chinese water spinach, which has wonderful crunchy edible stems, but you can use any greens from baby spinach to kale.

Makes 1 healthy serving

Ingredients:

1 tablespoon olive oil

1 teaspoon granulated garlic

¼ pound greens, roughly chopped

½ can spicy tomato juice or V8

2 farm fresh eggs

Sea salt and freshly ground pepper to taste

6–8 fresh basil leaves (or cilantro, parsley, fresh oregano, or dill)

Directions:

Heat a small sauté pan over medium-high heat and add the olive oil. Sprinkle in the granulated garlic and quickly follow with the greens. Cook just to wilt. Remove from pan and keep warm (I often just put them in the microwave so they don't chill too quickly to room temperature). Quickly add the tomato juice to the pan and bring to a simmer. Add the eggs and season with sea salt and pepper. Cover and simmer until the whites are solid but the yolks are still nice and runny (unless you like them harder). Remove the lid and sprinkle in the fresh herbs. Spoon on the plate with the greens and eat.

Chef's Diet Options:
Serve with sprouted-grain English muffins or whole-grain tortillas.
Add some diced summer squash or eggplant to the tomato juice before adding eggs.
Add your favorite chilies.
Splurge with some grated Parmesan or goat cheese.

129

Toasted or Grilled Whole-Grain Raisin Bread with Nut Butter and Stuff

Toast is probably the easiest breakfast you can make, unless you are a toast burner. I love a good sprouted-grain bread toasted extra crunchy and then turned into an open-faced sandwich to be eaten with a knife and fork. It makes it seem like more of a meal.

Makes 1 healthy serving

Ingredients:

2 slices favorite healthy whole-grain raisin bread

Nut butter—no additives, no added sugar—try crunchy peanut, sunflower, almond, cashew, soy nut, etc.

Sliced fruit, blueberries, banana, or peaches

Dried fruit, stewed figs, apricots, or prunes (cooked gently in water until plump and water turns syrupy)

Toasted seeds or nuts, pumpkins seeds, walnuts, sunflower seeds, almonds, pecans, etc.

Directions:

Toast bread to desired doneness. Spread with nut butter. Top with sliced fruit and spoon on stewed dried fruits. Finish with toasted nuts.

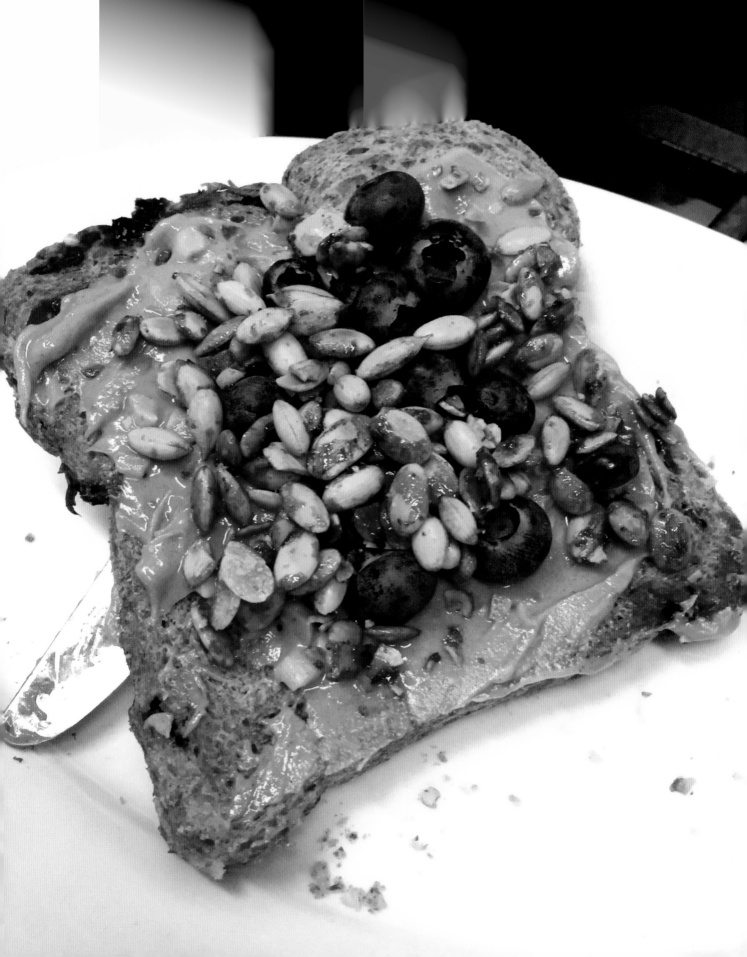

Stovetop "Baked" Eggs in Baked Sweet Potato Cups

If you are an Eggs & "Homies" kind of guy, you will like these eggs. It requires a little advance planning, so if you are making some baked sweet potatoes for dinner, throw in a few extras and keep them in the fridge for future use. Alternatively, you can now buy prewrapped sweet potatoes and cook them in just a few minutes in the microwave. I like to serve these with a crunchy green salad. A great dish to serve to a crowd on the weekend.

Makes 1 healthy serving

Ingredients:

1 tablespoon olive oil

1 small sweet potato, baked in the skin, cut in half, interior lightly smashed down to form a cup

2 cloves garlic, minced

2 farm fresh eggs

Rosemary sprigs

Sea salt and freshly cracked black pepper

2 tablespoons water

Optional: Nutritional yeast for sprinkling

Directions:

Heat oil in a small nonstick pan with a lid over medium-high heat. Add the sweet potato halves, skin-side down. Cook until the skin is crispy and crunchy, and add garlic. Crack an egg into each of the "cups." Season with salt and pepper and rosemary sprigs.

Lower temperature to medium and add water. Cook until whites are solid and yolks are runny. Remove lid, increase heat to medium high, and cook until garlic begins to smell nutty. Carefully transfer to warm plates. Sprinkle with nutritional yeast. Great served with a salad.

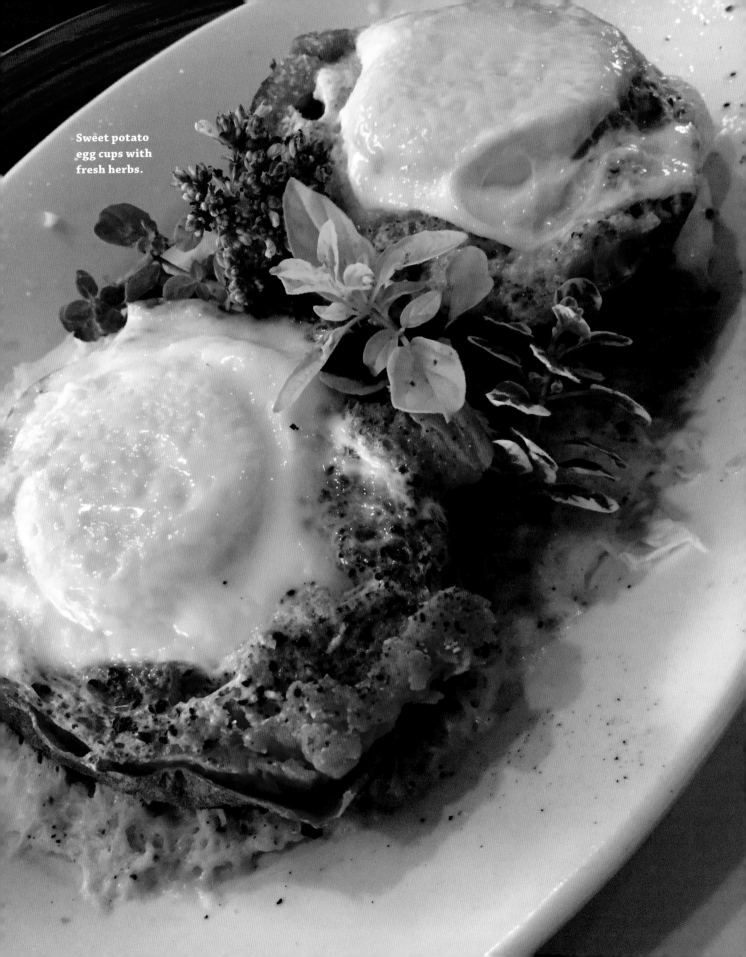

Sweet potato
egg cups with
fresh herbs.

Melon Berry Crunch

This quick, but complex, fruit breakfast gives you long-lasting energy with the combination of whole grains and dairy, slowing down the conversion of the fruit to sugar. You can doctor this recipe in many ways with a variety of ingredients.

Makes 1 healthy serving

Ingredients:

1 slice of a "personal"-sized watermelon

2 slices of cantaloupe

½ cup Greek yogurt

½ cup whole-grain, low-sugar cereal

6–8 blackberries

Favorite natural sweetener for drizzling

Directions:

Layer a slice of the watermelon on the plate with wedges of cantaloupe, yogurt, cereal, and berries. Drizzle with a touch of honey, agave syrup, or maple syrup.

Spiced Irish Oats with Agave, Berries, and Cream

Oatmeal is wonderful for scrubbing out our arteries and cleaning our pipes but I never met a bowl I liked until I discovered these Irish oats. They are available in cans at most supermarkets now and they are distinctly different from their cardboard-tube brethren. They are nutty, well textured, and toothsome. I make a big batch at a time so I can freeze servings in small bags for a quick morning meal without the 45-minute wait. You can also soak them overnight for a quicker preparation. Just read the can.

Makes 4 healthy servings

Ingredients:

1 ½ cups Irish steel-cut oats

4 cups water

½ teaspoon salt

¼ teaspoon ginger powder

¼ teaspoon ground cinnamon

¼ teaspoon ground nutmeg

¼ teaspoon ground allspice

2–3 turns black pepper

3 tablespoons agave nectar

Fat-free half-and-half as needed

½ pint fresh blueberries or blackberries

Directions:

Always cook oats in a heavy-bottomed saucepan so they don't burn. Rinse oats and drain well then place in saucepan. Add the remaining ingredients except the agave, half-and-half, and berries.

Bring to a boil and reduce heat to a simmer. Cook, stirring off and on for 45 minutes, until tender.

Taste and adjust seasoning as needed with agave. Serve in bowls with a little half-and-half, and top with blueberries or blackberries.

Chef's Diet Options:
Add toasted pine nuts or walnuts.
Add dried fruit like currants, raisins, or
  apricots.

LUNCHES

Lunch is often a meal that gets out of control. We are out of our homes and away from the structure that our homes give us. At work, stress is increased and support is lessened. It takes planning and focus to make follow-through a reality instead of a fantasy. Many of these dishes can be made ahead to take on the road with us. Most can be eaten cold or at room temperature, which makes them great for keeping in the office fridge or taking on a weekend picnic. One of the good things about this kind of cooking is that it is low in animal fats, which means reheating before eating isn't necessary. My general manager at FARMbloomington Restaurant, Ali, brings his "body builder buffet" to work every day so he isn't tempted by our "FARMfamous Parmesan and Garlic Fries," and he works in a restaurant! If you do eat out at lunch, remember to have a midmorning snack and drink a couple of glasses of water before you leave the office; it will cut your hunger and keep you from overordering. Choose lean proteins, whole grains, fresh salads, and veggies. Ask questions. Many dishes that sound healthy may have "secret ingredients" that might make them the wrong choice for you. Stay away from the allure of fried foods by ordering hummus or guacamole with veggie sticks for the table to share instead of French fries or a bread basket and butter. Sugary sodas and sweet tea are responsible for the majority of empty calories during the day. Make every day a spa day by creating a big, ice-cold container of cucumber and herb water for the office. I like adding a bit of kiwi, basil, and lime to mine. If you share your passion for a healthier lifestyle with your workmates, who knows—you might actually inspire others to do the same. Plant the seeds and watch them grow.

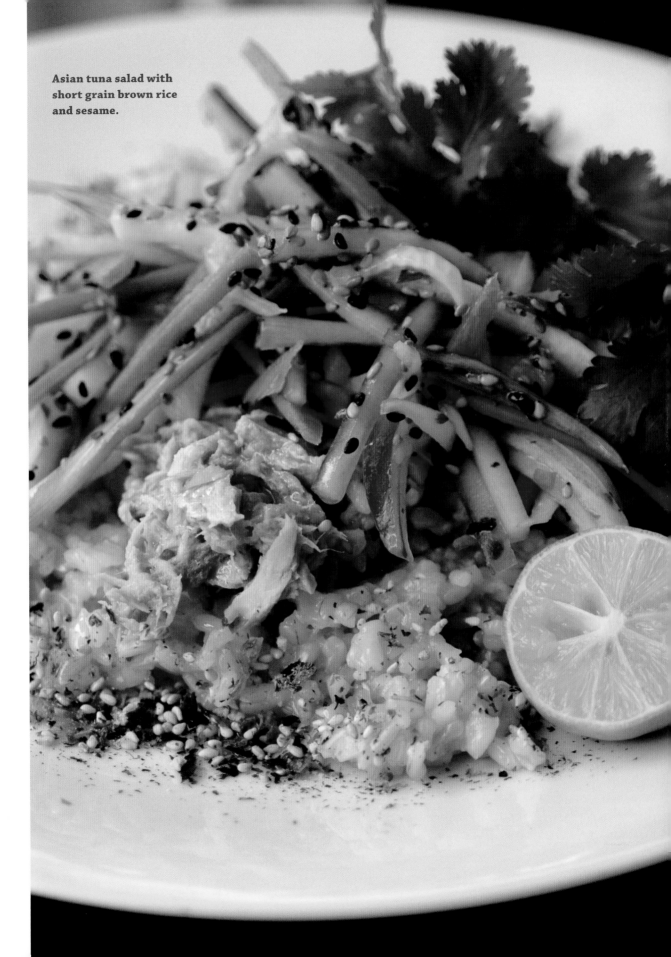

Asian tuna salad with short grain brown rice and sesame.

Beet and Pear Salad with Cabbage, Fennel, Feta, and Walnuts

This is a great side salad, but you could also have it as a main course lunch. It may sound like a lot of ingredients, but the flavors play well together. You can leave one or two out if you don't have everything in your fridge. Or, throw in that lonely radish or parsnip. No biggie. I like it with grilled or roasted meats, poultry, or fish. Throw leftovers in a whole wheat pita and your lunch tomorrow is ready.

Makes 4 healthy servings

Ingredients:

2 medium-sized beets, cooked, peeled, cut medium dice

1 pear (or apple) cored and diced medium

½ bulb fennel, shaved, tops reserved for garnish

1 small red onion, thinly sliced

½ head cabbage (Savoy, Napa, red, green, combo), cut chiffonade

½ cup toasted walnuts

½ cup feta cheese, diced medium

Juice of 1 lemon, 2 teaspoons zest

3 tablespoons extra-virgin olive oil (Note: EVOO is kitchen slang for extra-virgin olive oil)

Sea salt and freshly ground pepper to taste

Optional: 1 teaspoon fennel seeds, crushed with the back of a knife to release aroma and oils

Directions:

In a medium bowl, combine all ingredients and toss lightly. Allow to set 10–15 minutes to let the flavors meld. Taste and adjust seasoning with salt, pepper, additional lemon juice, and EVOO if needed. Best served at room temperature.

Bulgur, Cucumber, and Soy Salad with Sunflower Seeds and Citrus

This is one of my favorite salads. I like it spooned over a tangle of mixed greens as a main course salad, but you can use it as a side dish to dress up other meals as well. Serve it with grilled warm salmon or chicken or stuff it into cucumber cups to serve alongside chilled meat or fish. It is great in wraps or rolled in grape leaves, and it is a perfect healthy option to take to picnics and pitch-ins.

Makes 4 healthy servings

Ingredients:

1 cup bulger (roasted cracked wheat)

½ cucumber, diced

¼ cup sunflower kernels, toasted

1 pound, firm tofu, diced

2 scallions

½ cups fresh herbs (such as dill, cilantro, mint, parsley, or basil), roughly chopped

3 tablespoons extra-virgin olive oil

½ lemon, zested and juiced

Salt and pepper to taste

Mixed green salad as needed

Directions:

Rinse cracked wheat well and soak in 1 cup water for 1 to 1 ½ hours until tender. Drain off any excess water and toss with remaining ingredients. Season to taste. Serve with mixed greens.

Chef's Diet Options:
Add diced tomatoes.
Toss in some toasted almonds, pine nuts, or walnuts.
Spice it up with fresh chilies.
Add legumes like cooked green lentils or beans.

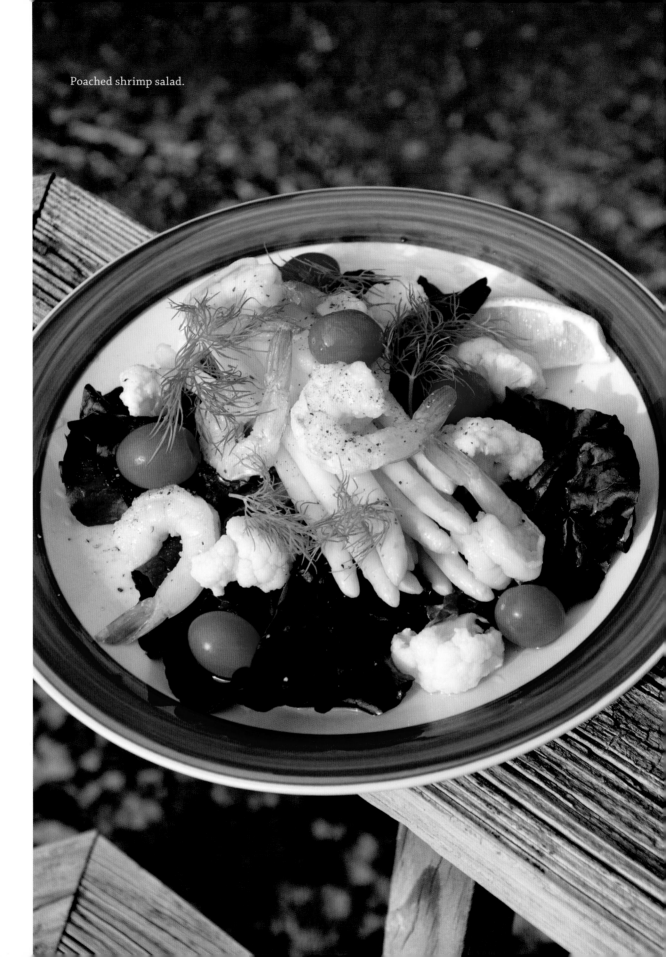

Poached shrimp salad.

Glass Noodles with Cucumbers, Garden Herbs, and Chili

Great as a side or as a main course luncheon salad. You can add grilled tuna, chicken breast, shrimp, or diced tofu. I love it served aside miso and mint marinated lamb.

Makes 4–6 healthy servings

Ingredients:

1 10.5 ounce package glass noodles (mung bean pasta)

¼ cup Thai fish sauce

¼ cup freshly squeezed lime juice, plus zest

¼ cup olive oil

3 tablespoon toasted sesame oil

2 tablespoon soy sauce

½ cup scallions, chopped

1 cucumber, julienned

½ cup daikon radish, diced

¼ cup chilies (or to taste), minced, use your favorite variety

1 cup herbs (combination of mint, Thai basil, and cilantro), chopped

½ cup black sesame or mixed sesame seeds

Salt and pepper to taste

Optional: Add tofu, edamame, snap peas, other vegetables, or grilled meats

Directions:

Cook noodles according to package directions and chill. Roughly chop and place in a large mixing bowl. Add remaining ingredients, and toss and season to taste.

141

Happy Mouth Quinoa Salad

This dish never disappoints. It is simple, yet complex, with the blending of sweet and savory. Great as a take-to-work lunch on its own or as a dance partner with your protein of choice. Mix it up and add whatever else you have around the house. No goji berries? Grapes! No walnuts? Almonds! No cilantro? Scallions! Keeps for 4–5 days in the fridge. Relax and enjoy.

Makes 4–6 healthy servings

Ingredients:

4 cups cooked quinoa (whatever color is available; I like the mixed colors)

1 apple, diced

½ medium cucumber, diced

¼ cup goji berries (or ½ cup raisins)

½ cup toasted walnuts

½ cup parsley or cilantro

3 tablespoons favorite light-colored vinegar (I like a good cider vinegar)

3 tablespoons good quality olive oil

Sea salt and freshly ground pepper to taste

Directions:

Put all ingredients in a medium-sized mixing bowl. Toss gently to combine. Taste and adjust seasoning with additional salt, pepper, and vinegar.

QUINOA YOU TELL ME THE TIME?

Although new to many in the United States, quinoa has been cultivated for 3,000 years in the Andes. The Incas called it the sacred seed, "the mother grain." Quinoa is high in protein, calcium, and iron. It is as close to a perfect food as exists in the vegetable or animal kingdoms.

The seeds are covered with a bitter resin-like coating called saponin. Unclean quinoa forms a soapy solution when mixed in water. To be edible, the saponin must be removed. Luckily most of the quinoa on the store shelves has had this laborious task completed, but it is always a good idea to give your quinoa a soak and a rinse just in case.

Japanese Tofu Salad with Shiitakes, Enokis, and Cucumbers

Westerners are a bit apprehensive about tofu. If they hear it is going to be served cold, they pretty much turn and run in fear. There is a reason I call it the "scary white stuff." Take a deep breath and give it a try. Nothing could be easier to prepare, and the contrast in textures is really very appealing. Tofu has a great protein punch and is low fat. As with all fermented soy products, the health benefits are numerous. Try it; you'll like it.

Makes 4 healthy servings

Ingredients:

½ cup shiitake mushrooms, thinly sliced (rehydrated dried mushrooms may be substituted)

1 package enoki mushrooms (woody base removed and mushrooms separated)

½ European cucumber, thinly sliced

1 small red onion, thinly sliced

3 tablespoons olive oil

2 tablespoons lemon juice

2 tablespoons soy sauce

1 clove garlic, minced

1 tablespoon ginger, minced

1 tablespoon Thai fish sauce

3 tablespoons sesame seeds (white, black, or mixed)

2 teaspoons sesame oil

1 container soft/silken tofu

Directions:

In a bowl, toss together the mushrooms, cucumber, and onions. Set aside until needed.

In another bowl, or a jar with a lid, combine the olive oil, lemon juice, soy sauce, garlic, ginger, fish sauce, sesame seeds, and oil. Whisk or shake to combine.

Slice the tofu in ¼-inch thick slices and arrange on plates or a platter. Dress the salad as needed, and spoon over and around tofu. Spoon any remaining dressing and sesame seeds over the tofu.

Chef's Diet Options:
Add some sliced radishes to the salad.
Blanch some thin string beans and add.
Spice it up with fresh or dried chilies to taste.
Steam the tofu and serve it warm with the vegetable salad.
Garnish with fresh herbs and edible flowers.

Vegan, Gluten-Free, Napa Cabbage "Tacos" with Spiced Walnut "Meat"

Makes 3–4 healthy servings

Ingredients:

For the walnut meat:

1 cup walnuts, toasted and cooled to room temperature

1 tablespoon chili powder

¼ teaspoon cayenne pepper

1 teaspoon granulated garlic

½ teaspoon cumin seeds

1 tablespoon extra-virgin olive oil

Salt and pepper to taste

Other ingredients needed:

1 head Napa cabbage (remove outer leaves and reserve for another use)

½ cup pico de gallo or your favorite salsa

1 avocado, diced

Optional: Cilantro, limes, and favorite hot sauce

Directions:

Place all walnut meat ingredients in food processor and pulse until roughly chopped. Set aside until needed (may be made up to a week in advance). Place Napa cabbage leaf "cups" on serving platter. Fill with spiced walnut meat, and top with pico de gallo, avocado, and cilantro. Accompany with limes and hot sauce.

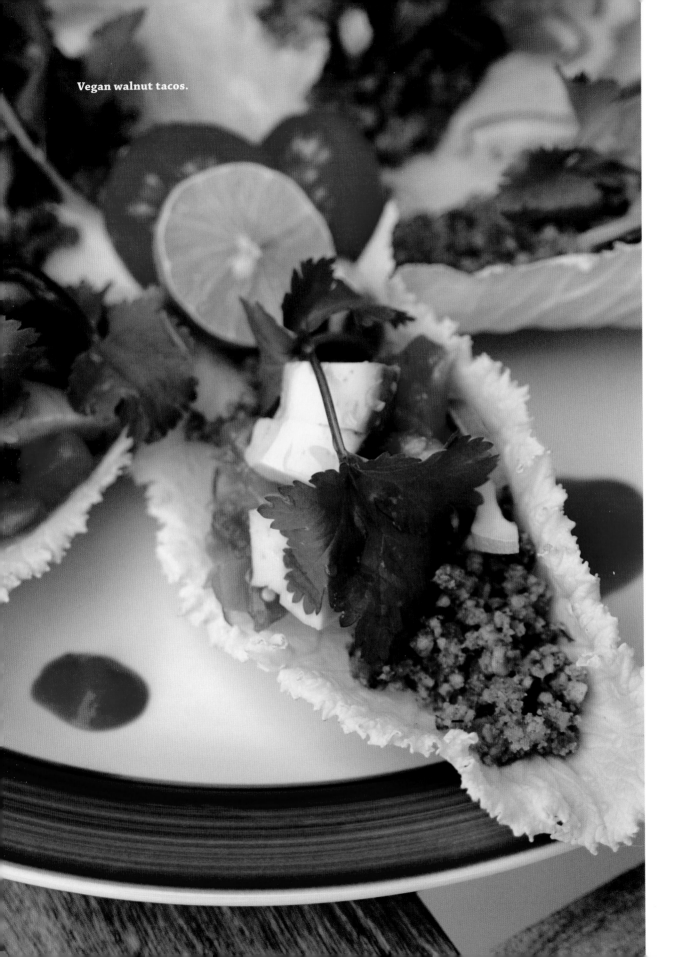
Vegan walnut tacos.

Lentils Salad with Fresh Herbs and Citrus

This is a master recipe to use for many hot or cold lentil dishes. Choose good-quality lentils such as lenticchie rodi from Italy or lentilles de Puy from France. Both have great earthy and meaty qualities to them and remain a bit more toothsome than typical American brown lentils, which tend to go mushy when cooked—a great quality if you are making a rich and hearty lentil soup but not so much for a salad.

Makes 6 healthy servings

Ingredients:

½ pound lentils (preferably French lentilles de Puy or Italian lenticchie rodi)

2 tablespoons olive oil

3 cloves garlic, minced

½ cup onions or shallots, minced

1 fresh bay leaf (or two dried)

1 sprig fresh thyme

5 black peppercorns, crushed

2 slices lemon (I use the two ends)

Water as needed

Salt and pepper to taste

Directions:

Wash the lentils to remove any dust. Remove any off-colored ones. Drain well.

Heat the olive oil in a medium heavy-bottomed saucepan and add the garlic. Cook until golden brown with a toasted aroma. Quickly add the onion and stir. Cook until soft.

Add the remaining ingredients and cover with water. Simmer until cooked tender but not mushy, adding additional water if needed. Do not add more water than needed or it will dilute the earthy flavors and your aromatic seasonings. Season to taste with salt and pepper. Spread in a glass baking dish and cool to room temperature. Refrigerate until needed.

Chef's Diet Options:
Toss with toasted walnuts, walnut oil, and citrus.

Mix with sun-dried tomatoes, capers, and Italian vinaigrette.

Add hearts of palm and cherry tomatoes and serve in lettuce hearts.

Mixed Greens with Black Quinoa

I love quinoa (pronounced *keenwa*). It is an extremely easy dish to cook and is so versatile. Here I serve it as a main dish with greens, but it also makes a great side dish with any grilled meat or fish or even a vegetable casserole. It is new to many people, so it is wonderful at a dinner party. Everyone will be impressed. I call for black quinoa, but you can use the more readily available white variety in its place. Leftover quinoa is great tossed with a vinaigrette and diced chicken or tofu or simply wrapped in a tortilla.

Bay Watch: It is worth going out of your way to find, or even better, grow, fresh bay leaves. We always keep four to five plants at the house and enjoy them year-round. In the spring, we put them outside and trim them way back, and they reward us with tasty foliage. Try them in stocks and sauces as well as pulverized in marinades and spice rubs. Whole leaves must be removed before serving. They are hard to swallow.

Makes 4 healthy servings

1 cup black quinoa (available at Whole Foods and other gourmet grocers); may substitute with white quinoa if the black is unavailable

1 tablespoon olive oil

3 cloves garlic, minced

1 small white onion, finely diced

1 bay leaf (fresh if available)

3–4 nice sprigs of fresh thyme or 1 teaspoon dried

Water as needed

Salt and pepper as needed

4 portions salad greens

Soak the quinoa in warm water for 10–15 minutes to remove any bitterness. Drain through a fine sieve and rinse well.

Heat the olive oil in a small saucepan and add the garlic. Cook until toasty and golden, and quickly add the onion. Sweat until soft and just starting to caramelize. Add the rinsed quinoa and herbs, and add water just to cover.

Bring to a boil and reduce to a simmer. Cook covered for approximately 15–20 minutes, adding additional water if needed.

Remove from heat and allow to sit covered for 10–15 minutes.

The quinoa should absorb any remaining water. If not, return to the heat and cook, stirring until all the liquid is absorbed. Season as needed with salt and pepper.

Serve warm or cold over greens of your choice.

Chef's Diet Options:
Add sliced tomatoes or avocado.
Add chopped fresh basil, cilantro, mint, parsley, or dill.
Stuff it into tomato or zucchini cups and bake.

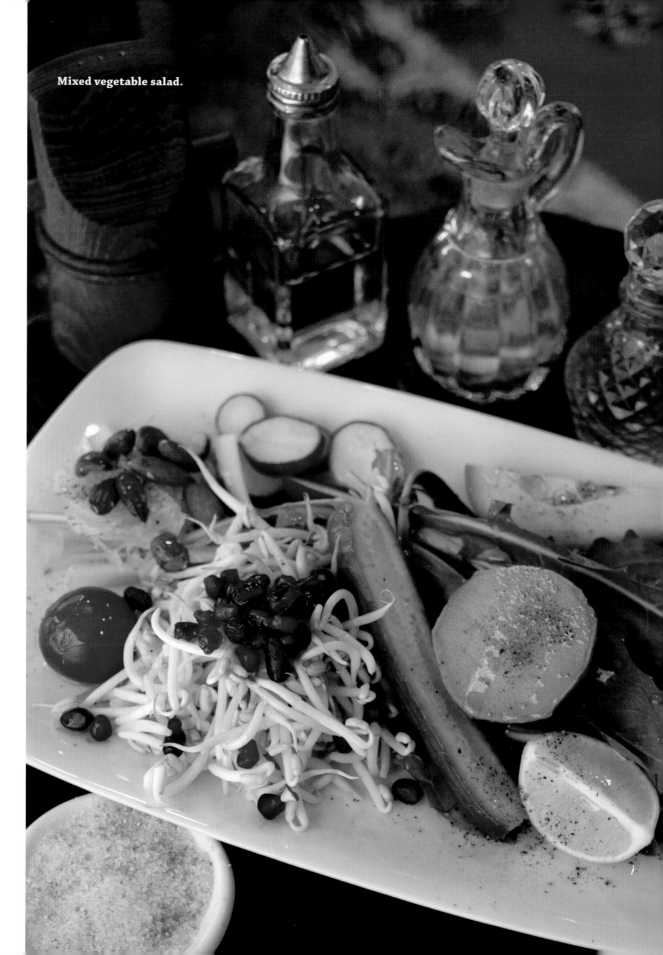

Mixed vegetable salad.

Tuna Salad with Avocado, Fresh Herbs, and Cherry Tomatoes

Keep some canned tuna around and you'll always have a quick meal at your fingertips. What you don't have to do is make it the way grandma did with mayo. Try this lighter, and tastier, version the next time you don't know what to have for lunch. Spoon it into a whole grain pita or serve with tahini brown rice or green salad. If you want to get fancy, plate it like I did with other salads in a stack and you'll amaze your friends.

There are many types of canned fish. Look for dolphin-safe varieties. If you are on a budget, any tuna is a good choice, but if you can afford water-packed chunk tuna, it is usually a more texturally pleasing choice. I love canned fish and always keep some around for a quick meal or snack.

Makes 2 healthy servings

Ingredients:

2 cans water-packed solid white tuna, reserve packing liquid

½ avocado, diced

½ small red onion, sliced as thinly as possible

6–8 cherry tomatoes (assorted colors if available), cut in halves

½ cup fresh herbs (whatever you have, parsley, dill, cilantro, chives, or a mix)

Juice of ½ lemon plus 2 teaspoons lemon zest

3 tablespoons good-quality extra-virgin olive oil

Sea salt, freshly ground pepper, and favorite hot sauce to taste

Directions:

In a medium sized mixing bowl, lightly flake tuna in packing liquid (it has flavor and nutrients!). Add remaining ingredients and toss gently to combine. Don't overmix—you want the tuna to remain slightly chunky. Adjust seasoning as you wish.

"Japanese" Tuna Fish Salad

Tuna fish salad gets a bad rap. Everyone secretly loves it but it has a bit of a lowbrow rep. I guess it is all the mayo. Well, I saw a can of imported red tuna from Italy that costs $25, so let's not be too judgmental. Tuna is a great protein source, and I always keep a few cans in the pantry for a postexercise minimeal. Although this recipe is a little more complicated than the traditional tuna salad, it really dresses up the dish and it is a great way to use tuna without dipping into the Miracle Whip.

Shiso is an herb used widely throughout Asia. It is a variety of mint that has a grassy, earthy flavor. One usually finds the green variety on sushi platters, but the darker purple sisters are easy to grow and actually will spread like wildfire in your garden. They are great in lettuce wraps and salads. Give shiso a try; it is available in most Asian markets.

Makes 4 healthy servings

Ingredients:

For the salad:

2 cans albacore tuna, chunk light variety

1 cup fresh bean sprouts (white mung bean preferable)

1 cup sliced shiitake (fresh or reconstituted) mushrooms

½ cup hijiki seaweed, soaked, rinsed and drained

½ medium white onion, thinly sliced

1 stalk celery, cut thin on a bias

For the dressing:

3 tablespoons olive oil

2 tablespoons soy sauce

1 tablespoon sesame oil

½ lemon, zested and juiced

1 tablespoon red wine vinegar

1 clove garlic, minced

1 tablespoon white sesame seeds

Freshly cracked black pepper to taste

Favorite salad greens as an accompaniment

Directions:

Drain the tuna gently so as not to squeeze all the moisture out of it. Carefully flake into nice pieces. Set aside.

Combine the remaining ingredients for the salad in a large bowl and toss. Mix ingredients for the dressing and adjust seasoning as needed. Toss the dressing with the salad ingredients to combine and fold in tuna chunks carefully. Serve with favorite salad greens such as mizuna or mesclun.

Chef's Diet Options:
Add chopped ginger to taste.
Add black sesame seeds.
Add chopped cilantro, mint, or scallions.
Toss with shredded Chinese cabbage.
Add thinly sliced or minced chili peppers.
Add bamboo shoots or sliced water chestnuts.
Use fresh tuna, grilled and diced.
Try with canned salmon.
Use other varieties of seaweed.

SOUPS

Call them whatever you want: velouté, potage, bisque, consommé, or chowder—this food is comforting, easy to eat, and great for making ahead. Soup can be the main attraction, or a starter for a more elaborate gathering. Soups are a great rainy day or long weekend project. They fill the room with nostalgic aromas of holidays and family and are easy to dish out to anyone who might stop by for a chat. Many soups freeze well and can be packed in individual or family-size containers for a quick meal. These recipes are great to use up seasonal bounty when the garden or farmers' market is overflowing. There is nothing like a warm bowl of soup when you are feeling under the weather, so remember that when a friend is feeling poorly. Soups are made for sharing, so make a big pot and take some over to that neighbor you haven't seen in a while or that older relative you have been meaning to visit. Not only will it make them feel better, but you will too.

Black Bean Soup

James Beard loved black bean soup. He thought it was one of the great American additions to New World cuisine.

Makes 8–10 healthy servings

Ingredients:

1 pound dried black beans

4 tablespoons olive oil

3 onions, chopped

1 green pepper, finely chopped

4 cloves garlic, minced

1 ham hock

Water as needed

2 tablespoons tomato paste

2 teaspoons cumin

2 teaspoons dried oregano

1 bay leaf

1 tablespoon salt

1 teaspoon black pepper

1 tablespoon vinegar or sherry

Directions:

Rinse the beans, and soak overnight in 4 quarts of water. Drain and set aside.

In a large pot, heat the olive oil. Add the onion, green pepper, and garlic and sauté over low heat for 10 minutes. Add beans and ham hock, and enough water to cover. Stir in tomato paste and seasoning (except for vinegar). Bring to a boil, cover, and simmer for 2 hours. Let cool slightly.

Remove half of the cooked beans, and using a blender, puree smooth. Return to pot. Add vinegar or sherry and stir well. Serve soup over white rice and top with fresh minced onion and fresh cilantro.

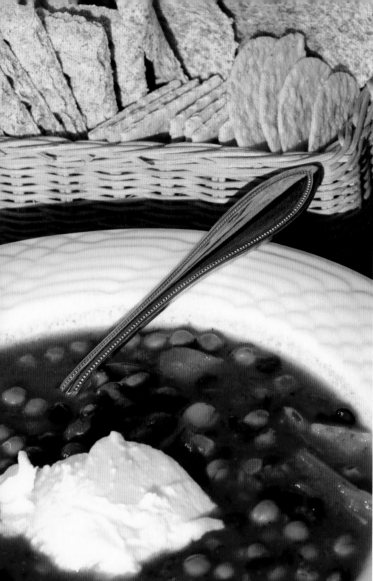

Bean soup.

Curry soup with coconut.

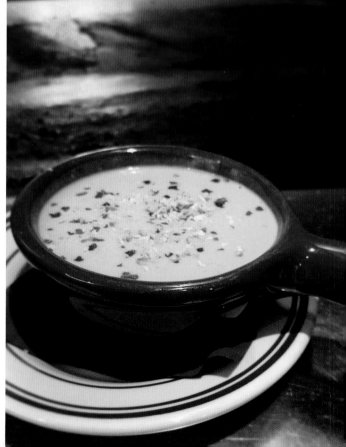

Butternut and Banana Bisque

I developed this dish when I was in the Caribbean. It has a wonderful balance of sweet and heat.

Makes 8–10 healthy servings

Ingredients:

¼ cup olive oil

2 Spanish onions

4 shallots

4 cloves garlic

1 tablespoon fresh ginger, minced

2 butternut squash (or similar amount of other hard squash or pumpkin)

1 ripe banana

1 green apple, peeled, cored, and roughly chopped

1 hot cherry pepper (available in Caribbean markets)

4 cups water (or light vegetable or chicken stock)

1 tablespoon kosher salt

1 tablespoon Anguillian Jerk Spice Rub (available on the website or in the spice section)

Juice of 1 lime

Salt and pepper to taste

Directions:

Heat a heavy-bottomed stainless steel pan over medium-high heat.

Drizzle in the olive oil and follow with the onions, shallots, garlic, and ginger. Reduce heat and sweat (cooking until tender but without coloring.) Peel the squash and discard the seeds and peels to the compost. Add the squash and the remaining ingredients except the lime and salt and pepper.

Return heat to high and bring to a boil, stirring often. Reduce heat to a simmer and cook until squash is tender. Remove cherry pepper (unless you like it spicier) and puree until very smooth in a blender.

Season to taste with the lime, salt, and pepper.

153

Chilled Beet Root Soup

Borscht is a classic Russian dish that should make its way onto every American menu from time to time.

Makes 8–10 healthy servings

Ingredients:

6 medium beets

3 bay leaves

3 tablespoons sea salt

1 tablespoon cracked black pepper

5 cloves

Water or chicken stock to cover

1 cup white vinegar

¼ cup olive oil

5 Spanish onions

10 large garlic cloves

4 good slices ginger (about ¼ cup chopped)

1 quart chicken stock

3 sprigs thyme (about 2 teaspoons dried)

¼ cup honey

¼ cup balsamic vinegar

Salt, pepper, and Tabasco to taste

Directions:

Place beets, bay leaves, salt, pepper, cloves, water, and vinegar in a large heavy-bottomed pot and bring to a boil over high heat. Simmer 1 to 1 ½ hours until very tender (when pierced with a fork). Chill under cold running water and peel. Set aside.

Heat olive oil in another large pan and sauté onions, garlic, and ginger until tender. Reduce heat and allow to caramelize evenly. Chop beets and add to pan along with the stock, thyme sprigs, honey, vinegar, and seasonings. Bring to a boil and reduce to a simmer. Cook until everything is tender (10–15 minutes).

Purée with hand blender or blender until smooth. Thin as needed with water. Adjust seasoning with salt, pepper, Tabasco, and additional vinegar as needed.

Chilled English Pea Soup with Mint

This is a favorite summertime soup for a lunch or as a starter for a weekend dinner. It is very classic and classy. Impress your bourgie friends with this one.

Makes 8–10 healthy servings

Ingredients:

2 tablespoons olive oil

1 medium onion, finely diced

2 cloves garlic, finely chopped

2 quarts light chicken stock (or water seasoned with bouillon)

2 pounds shelled fresh peas (frozen may be used in place)

2 teaspoons salt

1 teaspoon ginger powder

½ teaspoon ground white pepper (freshly ground preferred)

16 leaves fresh mint (cut chiffonade: fine), plus 6 nice tops

For garnish:

1 cup lightly whipped crème fraîche or heavy cream—leave liquid enough to spoon over soup

Cracked black pepper

Directions:

In a heavy-bottomed soup pot, add olive oil and gently cook the onions and garlic until tender but not brown. If needed, add a cup of the stock or water to retard browning. Add the chicken stock and bring to a boil.

Add peas and cook quickly over high heat until the starchy texture of peas becomes soft and the skins of the peas are tender. Add salt and spices, and chill quickly to room temperature in an ice bath. Puree in a blender until smooth and pass through a fine sieve. Add mint chiffonade.

To serve, ladle soup into chilled bowls and garnish with a swirl of cream, cracked black pepper, and mint sprigs. A little grated lemon zest is an optional additional garnish giving the soup a little fresh citrusy zip.

CHIFFONADE

Chiffonade is a classic culinary cut of leafy vegetables into thin ribbons. This usually allows the vegetable or herb to release its flavor while maintaining its texture and mouth feel.

Creamy Asparagus and Basil Soup with Soy

A light and healthy dish that travels well and is perfect for a healthy potluck.

Makes 8–10 healthy servings

Ingredients:

2 pounds asparagus (trim off 1 inch of bottom and discard into compost)

15 basil leaves

2 cloves garlic

½ jalapeño

2 tablespoons ginger

½ pound soft silken tofu

Cooking water from asparagus

Salt and pepper to taste

Directions:

Cut the asparagus stems in thin rounds and reserve the tips. Cover with just enough boiling water to cook and simmer until tender but not discolored. Place the asparagus in the basin of a blender and add remaining ingredients. Blend until smooth, and thin with cooking water as needed.

Boil asparagus tips in salted water for 2 minutes, chill under cold water, and reserve for garnish. Adjust seasoning and serve sprinkled with asparagus tips.

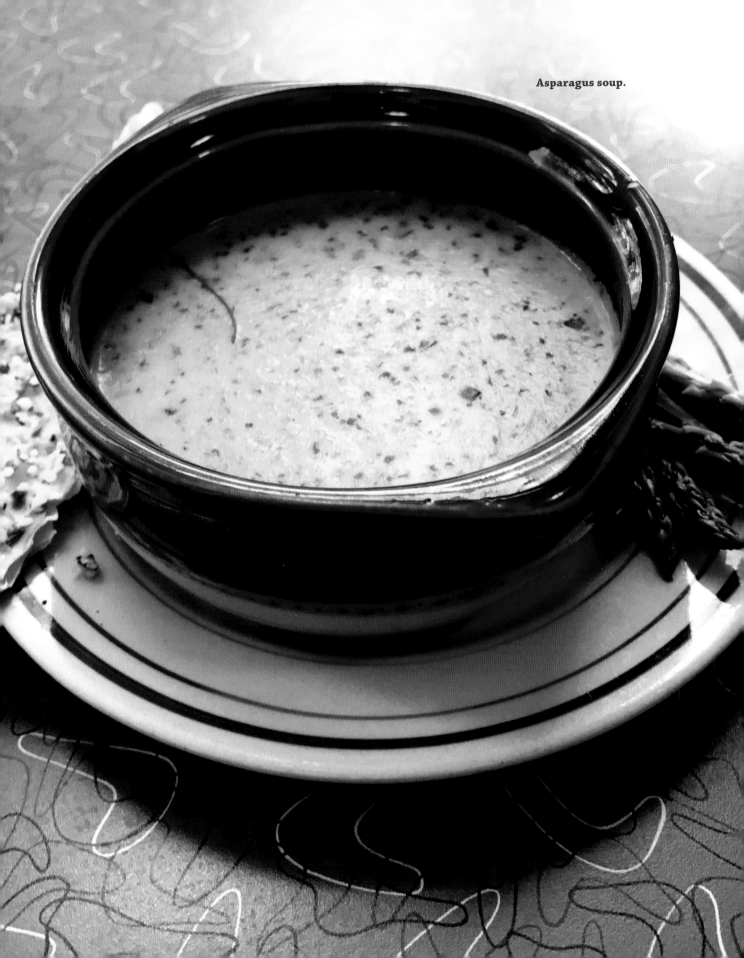

Asparagus soup.

A LITTLE SOMETHING ON THE SIDE

Side dishes have moved away from the supporting role and become the star of many menus both at restaurants and in the home. I know I get more excited about a dish of fresh-out-of-the-garden produce than I do about a piece of grilled tilapia! With the bounty of whole grains, greens, mushrooms, root vegetables, alliums, legumes, and such, how can you not get excited? Combining these ingredients in traditional or new and interesting ways is the great joy of cooking. Put together a few of these "side" dishes, and you have a wonderful main course. Make extra and many can be used as sandwich or salad ingredients for the next several days. Be creative and take the opportunity to make these recipes your own. For example, if you have a lonely parsnip in the salad crisper, chop it up and throw it in, you'll never know what will happen until you try. Don't let one ingredient keep you from making a dish; drop out any ingredients you don't like and try something else. Not a cilantro person? Try mint or basil.

Long Beans Braised with Stewed Tomatoes, Anchovies, and Pepper Flakes

Long beans are great for braising. They seem to retain their texture better than other green beans and almost get a meatiness to them. I love using homemade stewed tomatoes, but the canned variety will do in a pinch. These are also great served cold as a salad.

Makes 4–6 healthy servings

Ingredients:

2 tablespoons olive oil

4–5 cloves garlic, roughly chopped

6–8 anchovies, lightly crushed with their oil

½ teaspoon crushed red pepper flakes

2 pounds long beans, washed and trimmed, cut into two-inch lengths

2 cups stewed tomatoes

½ cups basil, roughly chopped

Salt and pepper to taste

Directions:

Heat the olive oil in a large sauté pan and add the garlic, anchovies, and chili flakes. Cook, stirring to release the flavors, and add the beans and stewed tomatoes. Cook until the liquids reduce and thicken and coat the beans. Add the basil and season with salt and pepper.

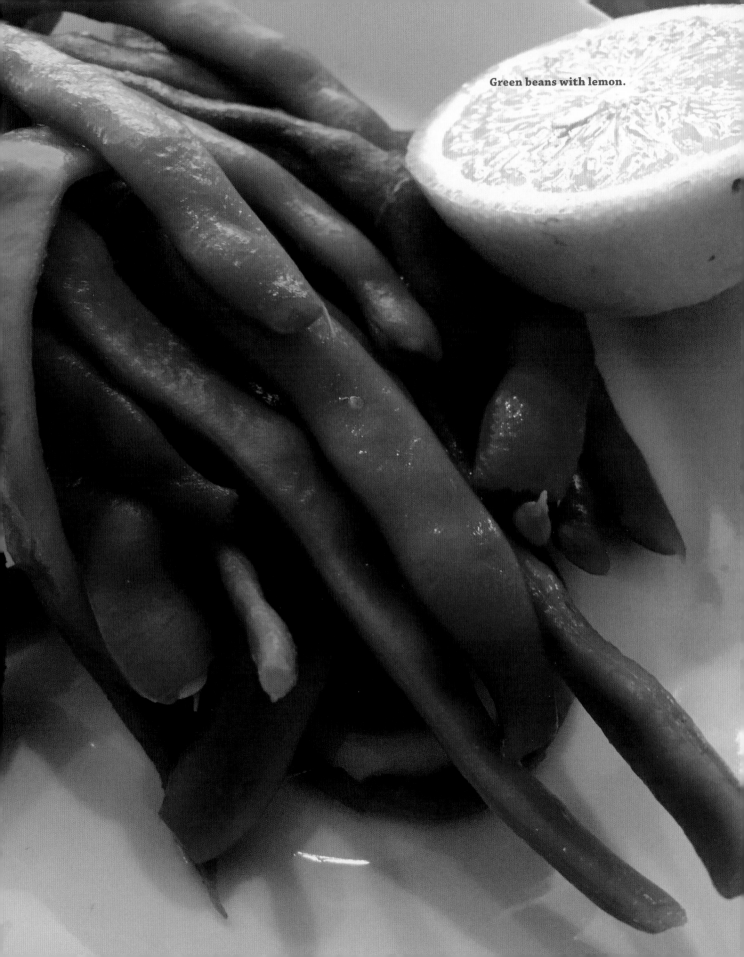
Green beans with lemon.

Asian Napa Cabbage and Carrot Slaw with Water Chestnuts and Sesame

This slaw will become a staple of your new regimen. Nice and crispy, it satisfies your need for crunch. It's great on its own, but is even better in a pita sandwich, topped with grilled chicken or a tempeh steak, or next to a burger.

Makes 4–6 healthy servings

Ingredients:

½ head Napa cabbage, shredded (or green, Savoy, bok choy, purple, or mixed cabbage)

1 large carrot, julienned

½ red onion, julienned

½ can water chestnuts

1 teaspoon toasted sesame oil

1 tablespoon olive oil

¼ cup tamari

Juice of ½ lemon or a whole lime

Sea salt and freshly ground pepper to taste

Optional: Chopped herbs such as scallions, Thai basil, cilantro, Asian garlic chive, or mixed herbs

Directions:

Place all ingredients in a medium bowl and toss. Season to taste.

Short-Grained Brown Rice with Tahini and Citrus

This is another staple in my fridge. It is so easy and so tasty you will keep it around all the time. The short-grained brown rice is very important. Regular brown rice seems to dry out and doesn't have the same nutty flavor or toothsome mouthfeel. This is great warm or cold as a side with about anything or just on top of greens. It is filling and satisfying. I know you'll love it.

Makes 4–6 healthy servings

Ingredients:

2 tablespoons tahini paste (ground sesame paste—store leftovers in the fridge)

¼ cup water

2 tablespoons lemon juice

2 teaspoons toasted sesame oil

4 cups cooked short-grained brown rice (follow recipe on package; I like to add a couple cloves of crushed garlic, minced onion, and chicken broth in place of water)

Sea salt, freshly ground pepper, and hot sauce to taste

Optional: Fresh herbs

Directions:

In a medium-sized mixing bowl, combine the tahini, water, lemon juice, and sesame oil. Whisk until smooth. Add brown rice (warm or cold, either is fine). Toss to combine and season to taste. Add chopped herbs if desired.

Regimen Cuisine Celery Root Mousseline

This recipe can be used in a variety of ways. It is great hot, right out of the blender, but also as an appetizer served chilled with some smoked salmon or even used as a dip or spread on sandwiches. Use it in 2–3 days. *Mousseline* is a French term used to describe a light and airy puree with lots of butter and cream. We re-create the mouthfeel without the fat.

Makes 2–4 healthy servings

Ingredients:

1 celery root (medium sized) peeled, rinsed, and cut in ½-inch dice

Pinch of salt

1 tablespoon lemon juice

Water as needed

½ cup Greek yogurt

¼ teaspoon mace

Knifepoint of cayenne

2 tablespoons best extra-virgin olive oil on hand

Salt and pepper to taste

Directions:

Place celery root, salt, and lemon juice in a heavy-bottomed saucepan. Add enough water to cook celery, but not too much. Bring to a boil and reduce heat to a simmer. Cook until celery is tender, stirring as needed. Strain celery, reserving any extra liquid.

Place yogurt and remaining ingredients in a high-powered blender (such as a Vitamix). Add the cooked celery and blend on low. Increase speed to high and blend until completely smooth, adding a little of the cooking liquid as needed. The puree should be thick and velvety like a rich French potato puree. Adjust seasoning as needed.

Spaghetti Squash Salad with Toasted Pumpkin Seeds and Citrus

Depending on the season, I use this both warm and cold as an accompaniment for any grilled, sautéed, or roasted fish or meat. Make sure you don't overcook the squash, you want it to have that nice crunchy texture. It's super simple, so don't mess it up!

You can toast the spaghetti squash seeds like you would toast pumpkin seeds at Halloween, or use pepitas (Mexican shelled green pumpkin seeds).

Makes 4–6 healthy servings (depending on the size of the squash)

Ingredients:

1 small to medium spaghetti squash—cook as directed (see Spaghetti Squash and Turkey and Quinoa Meatballs, p. 192)

Olive oil as needed

Lemon juice as needed

Chopped herbs

Sea salt and freshly ground pepper to taste

Toasted squash or pumpkin seeds

Directions:

Toss squash with seasonings and herbs. Taste and adjust seasoning. Sprinkle with seeds.

SNACK ATTACK

Snacking isn't a bad thing, in fact it can be a very good thing. It keeps our metabolism up as well as keeping folks from craving sweets, caffeine, and alcohol. It can also help you not overeat at the next meal. Next to drinking enough water, proper snacking can be one of the most important things you can do for yourself. Dr. K and I consider these "snacks" as your second and fourth small meal of the day. The key is eating the right things during these "minimeals." They should include high fiber and protein so you have a lower glycemic load. This will prolong energy without the "crash and burn" of a candy bar. Nuts and dried fruit are great. Try some low-fat string cheese or some turkey jerky. Bean dips or baba ghanoush (eggplant spread) and veggie sticks are great options. Cucumbers, radishes, and cherry tomatoes should be your friends. They are so easy to eat and full of both water and fiber. Remember to "eat your water" too! Figure out a few items you can carry with you or keep in the office fridge or desk drawer. Stay away from the vending machines, and you will become the master of your own universe.

Cauliflower "Popcorn"

Makes 4 healthy servings

Ingredients:

1 tablespoon extra-virgin olive oil

¼ teaspoon ground turmeric

Juice and zest of ½ lemon

2 tablespoons nutritional yeast

1 head cauliflower—washed and cut into small "popcorn-like" kernels

Kosher salt and freshly ground pepper to taste

Directions:

Place olive oil, turmeric, lemon juice and zest, and yeast in medium-size bowl, and mix to combine. Add cauliflower "popcorn" and toss well. Taste and adjust seasoning if needed. Serve in bowls and sprinkle with a little more nutritional yeast.

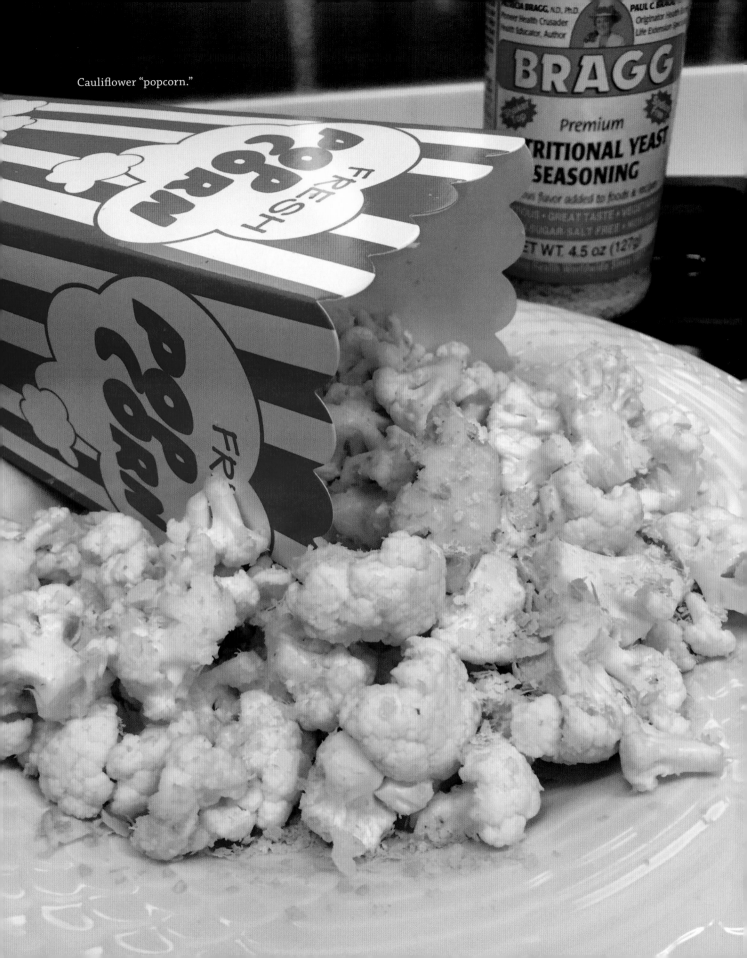

Cauliflower "popcorn."

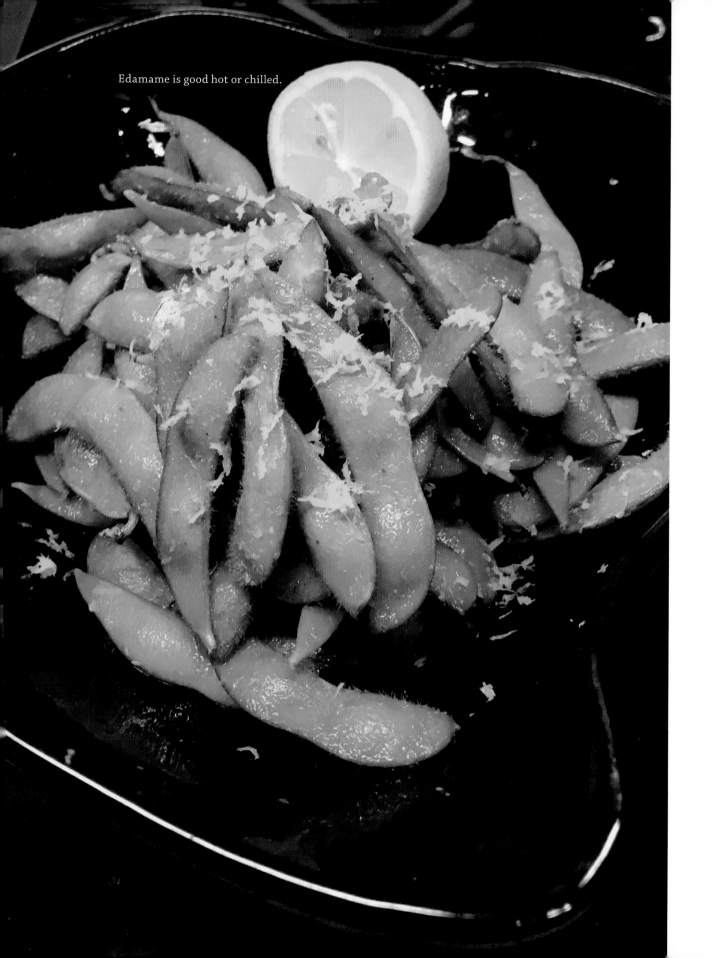

Edamame is good hot or chilled.

Steaming Soy

I love soybeans, a.k.a. edamame. They have become more and more available in grocery stores both shelled and in the pods. They are a classic Japanese bar snack and are best served simply. A lot of people have never had them cold, but they are excellent that way as well. They are kinda like eating a vegetarian version of New Orleans's crawdads, "pinch the tail and suck the head."

Makes 1 healthy serving

Ingredients:

8 ounces frozen edamame

2 teaspoons extra-virgin olive oil

Sea salt to taste

Aux Poivres Mixed Peppercorn Blend

Optional: Wedge of citrus

Directions:

Steam edamame until slightly softened. Toss in extra-virgin olive oil and season to taste. Serve immediately with a wedge of citrus.

Herbed Yogurt Dipping Sauce

This recipe is great as a dip, mayo replacement, or salad topping. I like to store it with a very thin coating of olive oil on top.

Makes 4 healthy servings

Ingredients:

1 cup Greek yogurt (or drained traditional
    yogurt)

1 tablespoon Greek Garlic Spice Blend

2 teaspoons Mediterranean Spice Blend

1 tablespoon extra-virgin olive oil

½ cup fresh herbs (such as scallions, parsley,
    chives, cilantro, mint, tarragon, etc.),
    chopped

Salt, pepper, and hot sauce to taste

Directions:

Mix ingredients and allow to sit at least 15 minutes—overnight is even better. Store in refrigerator for up to a week.

Sweet Cherries and Yogurt Dip

Makes 1 healthy serving

Ingredients:

8 ounces cherry tomatoes, multicolored

2 ounces herbed yogurt dipping sauce
   (see recipe above)

Minty Pea Guacamole

This is a favorite of mine and is great for many uses. Replace mayo with it on sandwiches and pita pockets, use it as a dip, use it on salads, use it as a sauce! You don't even have to tell your family and friends there is tofu in it! Make a batch and use it within 3–4 days.

Makes 4–6 healthy servings

Ingredients:

1 pound sweet green peas, blanched until skins
   are tender then shocked in ice water

1 chili pepper (jalapeño or your favorite
   depending on how hot you like it), roughly
   chopped

1 tablespoon ginger, minced

½ cup mint leaves

½ pound silken tofu

½ cup olive oil

Salt and pepper to taste

Tabasco as needed

Directions:

Puree ingredients together in a food processor or blender until smooth. Season to taste with salt, pepper, and Tabasco.

Orange Lentil Spread

This is a great "vegetable pâté," to spread on rice crackers or use as a dip for crudités; it is also good on lettuce "wraps" and veggie plates and can be eaten hot or cold. It is kinda like a hummus, but lentils cook much quicker and they practically puree themselves, so you don't have to break out the blender or food processor.

Makes 4–6 healthy servings

Ingredients:

½ pound orange or yellow lentils

1 Spanish onion

3 cloves garlic

¼ cup olive oil

2 cups water

1 tablespoon Kitchen D'Orr Spice Blend

Juice of 1 lemon, plus 2 teaspoons zest

Sea salt and freshly ground pepper to taste

Favorite hot sauce to taste

Directions:

Pick through and wash lentils, and set aside. Finely mince onions and garlic and sauté in olive oil until tender in a medium-sized soup pot.

Add lentils and water and bring to a boil. Skim off impurities. Add desired seasonings and cook until lentils are tender and starting to crumble and fall apart. Reduce heat and cook, stirring often, until it reaches a "hummusy" thickness. Season to taste with lemon, salt, pepper, and hot sauce.

Eat hot, or chill until needed. Keep up to 7 days in the fridge.

SMART SIPS

Since bodies are over 50 percent water, keeping liquids in balance is important. The leaner the body, the higher the percentage of water we contain. Water is the most important part of our diet. In fact, you would typically die from thirst before hunger. Water is calorie free and helps reduce hunger by combining with fiber and keeping you feeling satiated. Find a good, healthy, clean source for water and drink as much as you can. It is good to have a filter for your water in your home to keep toxins and impurities out of your glass. Stay away from drinks that are highly processed or contain ingredients from the evil empire, such as corn syrup, artificial sweeteners, and white sugar. Processed fruit juices are often almost as bad as sweetened drinks because most of the fiber and some of the antioxidants and nutrients have been depleted.

Water can become boring, but there are tons of ways to make it more exciting. If you have ever been to an expensive spa, you probably have enjoyed cucumber, mint, or citrus water from a pretty glass decanter. These naturally flavored waters are not only refreshing; they are also naturally cooling drinks through their liquidity, aromas, and antioxidant-rich ingredients. At home you can prepare "mocktails" with sparkling water, fruit juices, citrus, herbs, and fresh fruit garnishes. Try a craft tonic water with kumquat slices and bruised mint leaves; sparkling water with pure pomegranate juice, lime, and agave; or iced green tea sweetened with honeydew juice and lemon. How about iced turmeric and ginger tea with honey? If you have an herb garden, try making mint ice cubes and using edible herb and garden flowers to float on top of your summertime drinks for a playful tropical feel.

During the cooler months, you might want warmer drinks like herbal teas, warm unfiltered cider with ginger and spices, turmeric golden soy milk, or hot chocolate made with coconut milk, cinnamon, cayenne, and cocoa. Many of these can be made ahead and kept hot in a thermos for several hours. Homemade chai tea is another option. The spices are wonderfully warming and have many beneficial qualities. Warm apple juice with sage, honey, and citrus is another unusual warm beverage you can share with family and friends when you take a break from shoveling snow on that cold January day. Dr. K loves to can tomato juice during the summer, and there is nothing better on a frigid day than a mug of hot, spicy homemade tomato juice with black pepper, garlic powder, and a dash of cayenne.

We also suggest that you branch out a bit on your beverages. Try some kombucha, the antioxidant-rich probiotic fermented tea that is available in many flavors like ginger, hibiscus, berry, or traditional. Chef D likes the one with chia seeds added to it. Kvass is a traditional beer-like drink from Poland and Russia traditionally made with fermented bread. A healthier borscht-like beet version is available at our local food co-op and it, too, is available with different flavorings like kimchi and chili pepper. Kvass has a bold deep purple color and when poured into a wine glass looks like . . . well . . . wine. Both of these beverages are good cocktail hour stand-ins and pair well with many foods.

Yes, there are a ton of options when it comes to the MyTendWell philosophy, but we always suggest that you quench your thirst with plenty of water, then drink all other beverages for enjoyment and pleasure. Start and finish your day with a large glass or two of H$_2$O and you'll find yourself refreshed, cleansed, and satisfied. Drink up!

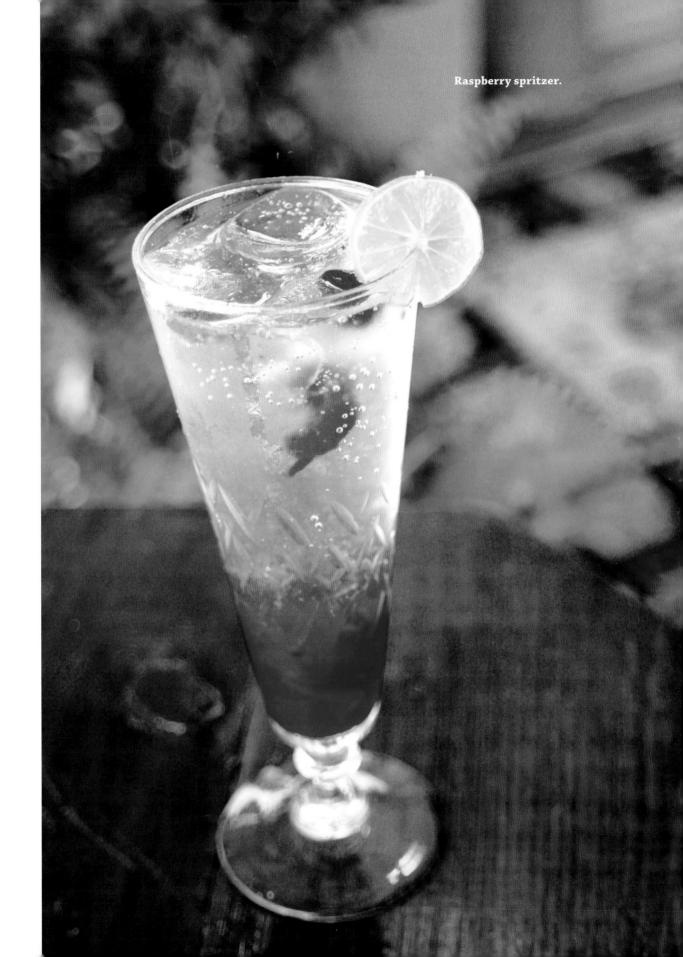

Raspberry spritzer.

Agave Aperitif with Raspberry and Key Lime

This is a great, light, fizzy drink that you can vary with ingredients, seasons, and your own inspiration. Add some mint, verbena, or rosemary sprigs. Change up the berries with peaches or agave for honey or maple syrup. Honey does harden when chilled, so mix it with the citrus juice before adding the ice and chilled soda water.

Makes 2 healthy servings

Ingredients:

2 tablespoons agave

8–10 raspberries

Juice of 2 key limes, plus wedges for garnish

16 ounces of club soda

Ice

Directions:

Choose two nice tall glasses and, in each, place 1 tablespoon agave, 3–4 raspberries, and the juice of 1 key lime. Muddle the fruit and citrus lightly and fill glass with ice. Top with soda water and garnish with a couple more raspberries and lime wedges.

Mellow Yellow Iced Tea

Sometimes you just need to chill out and get mellow; this light beverage will help get you there. This is a less-rich version of the MyTendWell Golden Milk above. Make a double or triple batch and store in the fridge. If you have a sunny patio, you can also brew this as a sun tea.

Makes 2 healthy servings

Ingredients:

2 cups water

1 inch fresh ginger root, grated on microplane

2 inches fresh turmeric root, grated on microplane

¼ cup honey

1 pinch of salt

2 green tea bags

Optional: A handful of fresh mint leaves, favorite citrus wedges, and juice

Directions:

Bring water to a boil and add minced ginger, turmeric, honey, and salt. Simmer covered for 5–10 minutes then turn off the heat. Add the green tea bag and mint if desired and steep for 3 minutes. Strain out the solids using a fine mesh strainer and chill.

Fill two glasses with ice cubes and pour the tea over. Add fresh citrus juice and honey to taste, garnish with sliced citrus and mint sprigs.

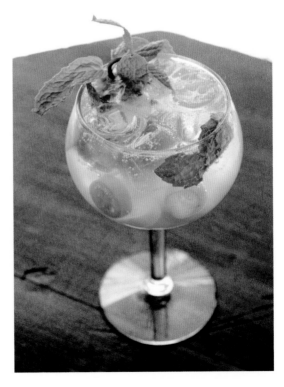

Kumquat mint sparkle.

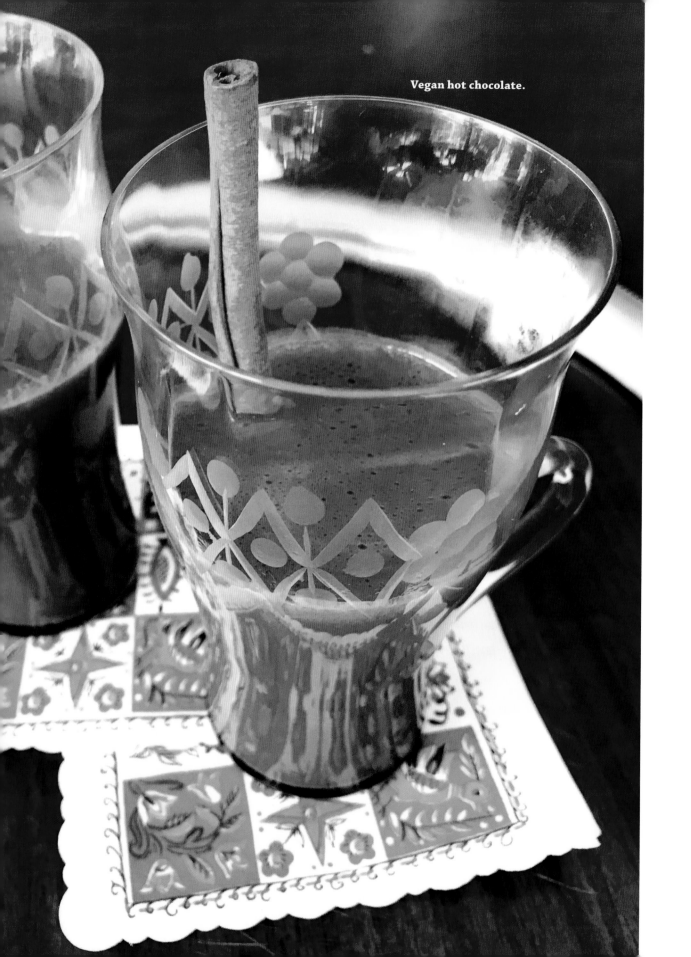

Vegan hot chocolate.

Chef D's Coconut Milk Mexican Hot Chocolate

A cup of hot cocoa always takes me back to my childhood memories. We would be sledding down the hill in the backyard or out on the frozen lake playing hockey or ice fishing, and Mom would be inside making hot chocolate and treats of some kind. Those are warm and comforting memories from when I was too young to have had much bad stuff happen to me. This recipe is vegan, but tastes as rich and decadent as any other I've had. It is lightly sweetened with agave, but I like it fairly bitter from the unsweetened chocolate and cocoa powder. Chocolate is full of phytonutrients and flavonoids, so it aids in removing free radicals from your body. Oh, and it tastes sexy as hell!

Note: By mistake, Chef D discovered that when chilled, this drink makes a mousse that is a velvety flavor bomb!

Makes 2 very rich and healthy small cups

Ingredients:

1 can unsweetened coconut milk

½ cup cocoa powder

1 tablespoon agave syrup

½ teaspoon cinnamon

1 knife's point ground allspice

1 knife's point cayenne pepper

½ cup water

2 squares Ghirardelli 100 percent unsweetened chocolate, chopped

Optional: Large cinnamon sticks for stirring

Directions:

Combine coconut milk, cocoa, agave, spices, and water in a small saucepan. Whisk lightly to incorporate ingredients. Bring to a simmer and allow to cook 4–5 minutes without boiling. When coconut milk is hot, remove from heat and whisk in the chocolate.

Pour into a quart-sized Plexiglas measuring cup, and blend with a handheld immersion blender (or just pour in the basin of a traditional blender) until smooth and frothy.

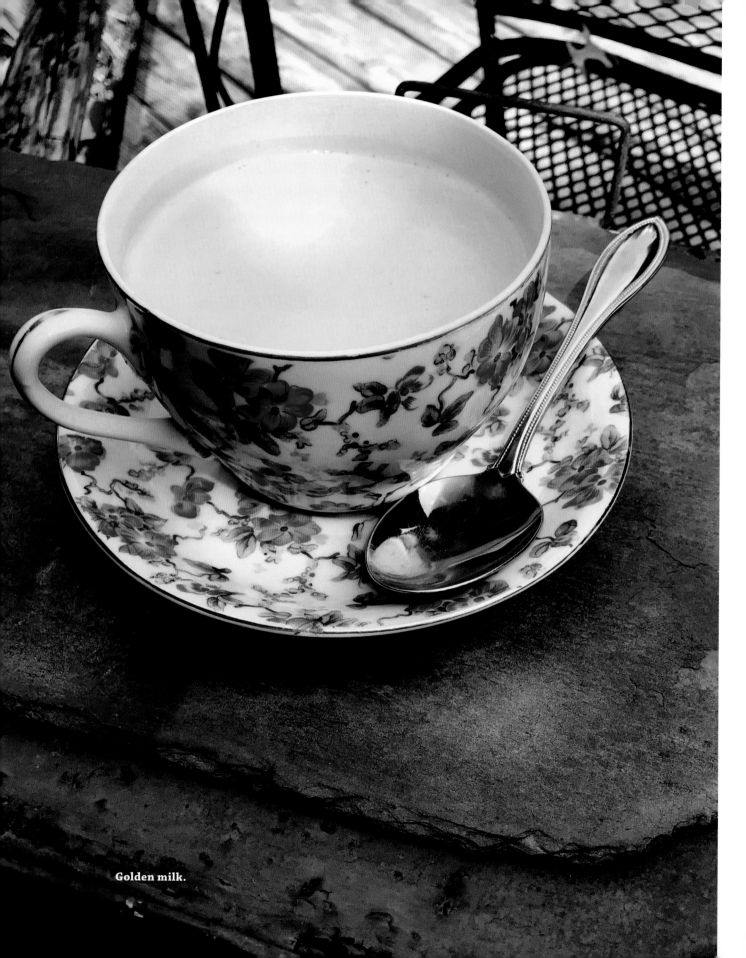

Golden milk.

MyTendWell Golden Milk

Turmeric is currently the darling of the healthy food movement. Recent studies have shown some evidence that turmeric can reduce inflammation and support brain and joint health. It has also been shown that when combined with healthy fats and black peppercorns, the alkaloid piperine absorption is taken to the max! With the addition of freshly grated ginger, you will not only get help with arthritis, bursitis, and other musculoskeletal ailments, but this drink can also calm digestive issues and assist in healthy sleep.

Note: Turmeric stains badly, especially fresh, so avoid doing this on white countertops or wearing white clothes. A spritz of all-purpose cleaner should solve the problem, though.

Makes 2 healthy servings

Ingredients:

2 cups of your favorite vegan "milk" such as soy, almond, hemp, or coconut

½ tablespoon fresh ginger, peeled and grated

1 tablespoon fresh turmeric, peeled and grated

3–4 black peppercorns, crushed

2–3 cardamom pods, crushed with the back of a knife

2–3 strips of lemon peel

Knifepoint of cayenne pepper

Optional: 2 tablespoons unfiltered honey (or agave or maple syrup), or to taste

Directions:

Heat all ingredients in a small saucepan and stir well. Bring to a simmer and simmer covered for 10 minutes. Blend with a handheld immersion blender. Strain and sweeten to taste (if desired).

Cranberry, Meyer Lemon, and Tonic

Cranberries are wonderfully sour and make you pucker. They are also great for your bladder. You can use fresh ones, which will float and make a pretty garnish, but thawed frozen berries work very well and are easier to muddle. Meyer lemons are sweeter than normal lemons, and you can even eat their peels if they are organic. Again, change it up and make it your own. Our recipes are only guidelines and inspiration. Have fun.

Makes 2 healthy servings

Ingredients:

2 tablespoons maple syrup

10–12 frozen cranberries, thawed, plus more for garnish or fresh ones for garnish

½ cup 100 percent cranberry juice

Juice of a Meyer lemon, plus wedges for garnish

Ice

16 ounces of tonic water (I use diet usually, or a nice craft one if I can find it)

Directions:

In a glass pitcher, combine the maple syrup, berries, cranberry juice, and lemon juice. Muddle to combine and fill with ice. Pour over tonic and lightly stir. Serve in glasses garnished with Meyer lemon wedges and a few more fresh or frozen cranberries.

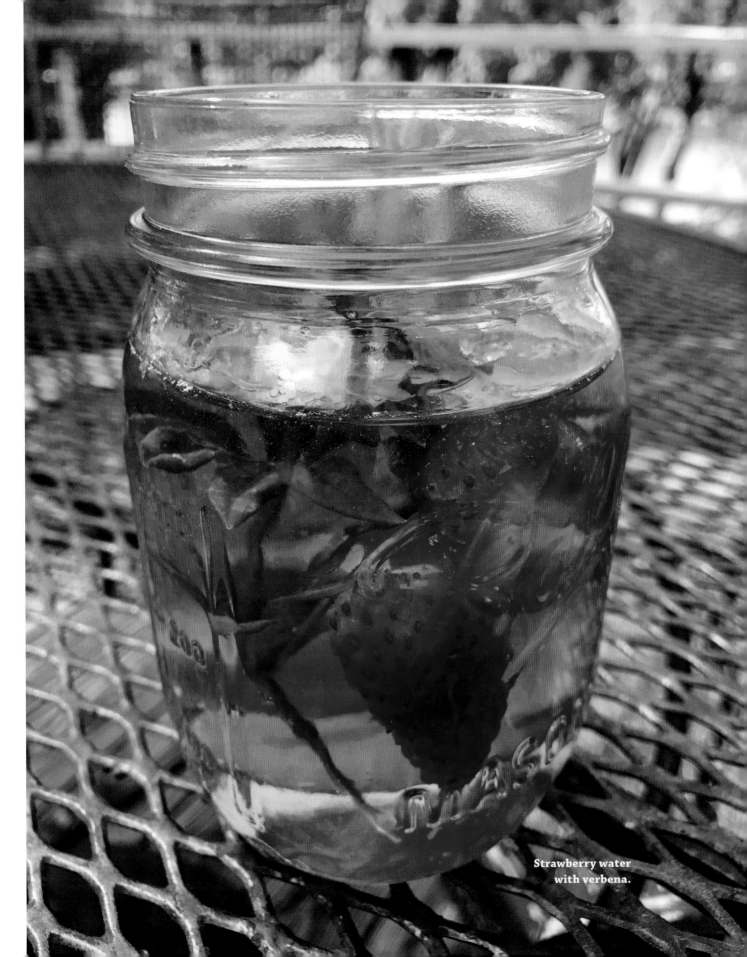

Strawberry water
with verbena.

DINNERS

Dinner is a time to share—your day and your accomplishments, your successes and failures, your fears and worries. Most of all, however, it's a time to share food and the enjoyable task of putting it on the table. These meals may take a little longer to shop for and prepare but that can be thought of as part of the fun. Surround yourself with people who love to cook and eat, and you will be a happier person. Remember that you must always keep a sense of childlike interest and playfulness in everything you do. Laugh at your kitchen disasters and celebrate your achievements. You often can't really pick who you are going to have a business lunch with, but at dinnertime you can gather those you truly enjoy into the kitchen and spend some quality time. Remember to share tasks and ask for help, and whoever does the cooking doesn't have to clean up!

Unilateral Grilled Salmon with Citrus and Spice

Many people are scared to cook fish on the grill. This recipe is basically foolproof. I usually use a gas grill for this, but if you are using a charcoal grill, build the fire on one side and cook the fish on the other. Salmon is perfect for this recipe because of its fattiness, but you can experiment with other fish as well.

Makes 4 healthy servings

Ingredients:

2 pounds salmon fillet (thick-cut)

1 ½ tablespoons olive oil

1 lemon, zest and juice

2 teaspoon Kitchen D'Orr Spice Blend

1 teaspoon black peppercorns, crushed

4 cloves garlic, minced

1 tablespoon lemon thyme, roughly chopped

Course sea salt as needed

Optional: Lemon wedges and olive oil for drizzling

Directions:

Cut salmon fillet into 4 equal pieces. Set the fillets in a baking dish skin side down. Combine the remaining ingredients in a small bowl and mix to form a paste. Rub this paste evenly on the exposed side of the salmon and refrigerate for 1 hour.

While the salmon is marinating, heat the grill to high heat. When hot, place the salmon on the grill, close cover, and turn off the gas. Cook for 7–10 minutes until medium rare. Remove with a wide spatula to serving dish, sprinkle with sea salt, and drizzle with olive oil and lemon juice.

Chef's Diet Options:
Try halibut or thick turbot steaks.
Add some fresh chilies to the wet rub.
Add curry or turmeric to the rub.
Serve over sliced tomatoes or roasted beet salad.
Serve with sautéed kale.

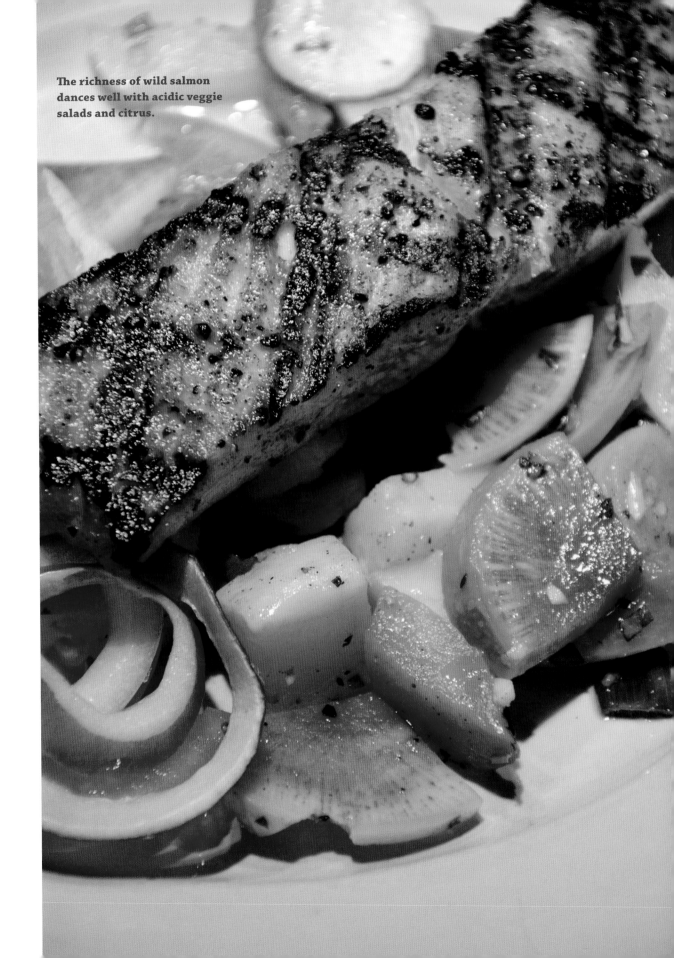

The richness of wild salmon dances well with acidic veggie salads and citrus.

Chef's Diet Fry-Pan Meatloaf

I love this dish that came to being because of some leftover oatmeal. It is typical to add white bread soaked in milk or breadcrumbs to classic meatloaf. The oatmeal does an even better job keeping the recipe moist as well as giving it great texture. I like using a Teflon pan to cook the meatloaf. It gives a unique round presentation, you don't have to worry about it sticking, and it is easy to clean up afterward. The dish is amazing served hot but makes great "pâté-like" slices served cold with a big salad for lunch. I've even grilled the chilled slices and served them like gyros with sprouts, hummus, and whole wheat pita bread.

Makes 4–6 healthy servings

Ingredients:

1 ½ pounds ground lean turkey or chicken

2 eggs

1 cup leftover cooked oatmeal, preferably Irish steel-cut variety (chilled)

1 can (8 ounces) spicy tomato sauce (I like Goya brand)

1 rib celery, diced small

1 onion, finely diced

4 cloves garlic, minced

1 tablespoon dried fines herbes (like Mediterranean blend or herbes de Provence)

1 teaspoon Chinese five spice (or Kitchen D'Orr Spice Blend)

1 teaspoon salt

1 teaspoon freshly ground pepper

Olive oil spray as needed

Directions:

Preheat oven to 350 degrees. Mix all ingredients well and chill until needed. Cook a small amount and taste for seasoning. Adjust as needed. When oven is hot, place a 10-inch nonstick sauté pan with an ovenproof handle over medium-high heat until hot. Spray with olive oil spray.

Add the mixture to the pan and form into a round loaf with a wooden spoon or spatula. Place in the oven and cook for 45 minutes to 1 hour or until juices run clear when poked in the center with knife. Remove from oven and allow to rest at least 25 minutes before serving. Accompany with cauliflower puree, steamed green beans, or asparagus.

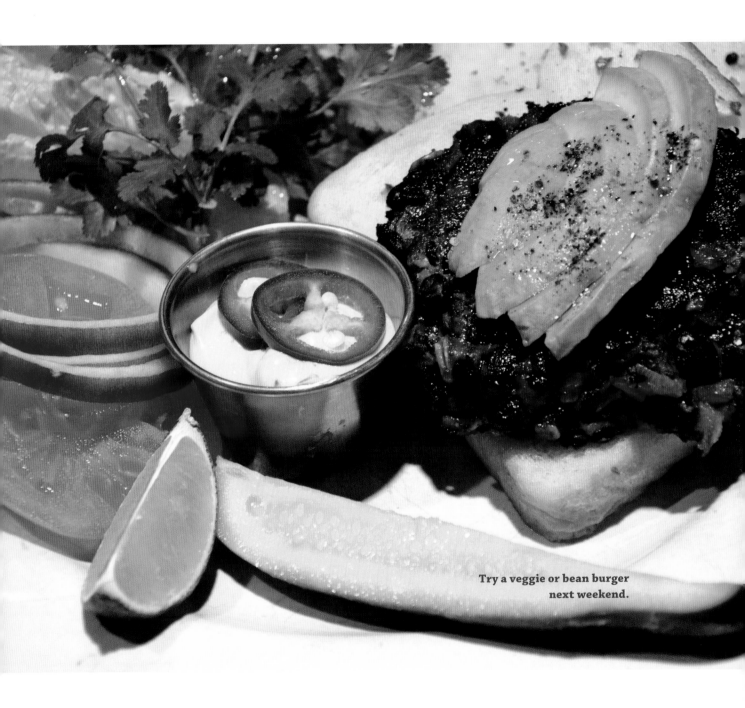

Try a veggie or bean burger next weekend.

Fisherman's Catch in Tamarind Glaze

I used this glaze to perk up grouper, which tends to want the extra zing that tamarind has. Adding the Thai fish sauce makes it a bit Asian, so I like to serve this with quickly sautéed bok choy. You'll also love it over pork, chicken, or game birds.

Makes 4 healthy servings

Ingredients:

4 5-ounce portions of your favorite fish fillet

Salt and pepper

For the glaze:

2 tablespoons tamarind paste (seeds removed)

2 tablespoons Thai fish sauce

1 tablespoon fresh ginger, minced

1 tablespoon garlic, minced

3 tablespoons honey

3 tablespoons dark molasses

2 tablespoons ketchup

2 tablespoons fresh lime juice

1 teaspoon freshly ground black pepper

1 tablespoon Kitchen D'Orr Aux Poivres Spice Blend

1 tablespoon Kitchen D'Orr Spice Blend

Directions:

In the bowl of a food processor or blender, combine the tamarind paste, fish sauce, ginger, garlic, honey, molasses, ketchup, lime juice, pepper, and the Aux Poivres and Kitchen D'Orr spice blends until smooth. Pour into a saucepan and bring to a boil. Remove from heat and place in a storage container. Refrigerate until needed.

To use, simply marinate the fish fillet in a tablespoon or so of glaze for 20–30 minutes, and then broil until just translucent in the center. Remove from oven and serve over your favorite stir-fried veggies. Drizzle with a little more glaze.

Tuscan Flatiron Steak with Garlic, Rosemary, and Lemon

I love the classic Italian flavors of garlic and rosemary with meat, and this dish uses them deliciously. It is a simple grilled dish served with wedges of lemon and a drizzle of good olive oil, as is done in Florence. I love it done on an outdoor grill, but I've used a Teflon grill pan with great results as well. Don't forget to let the steak rest after you take it off the grill. I like to rest meat for about the same amount of time as I cook it. The result is beautifully rosy and tender meat that holds its moisture in.

Makes 4 healthy servings

Ingredients:

1 ½ pounds flatiron steak

3 cloves garlic

2 tablespoons fresh rosemary

2 tablespoons olive oil (extra for drizzling)

Crushed black pepper as needed

Sea salt as needed

Olive oil spray as needed

1 lemon, cut into wedges

Directions:

Butterfly the steak and rub the interior with the chopped garlic, rosemary, olive oil, and cracked black pepper. Refrigerate until 15 minutes before cooking. When meat is at room temperature rub with a little olive oil and season with sea salt and additional cracked pepper.

Preheat grill or grill pan until very hot. Spray grill or grill pan with a little olive oil spray. Place flatiron steak uncut side down and grill for 5–7 minutes until well marked. Reduce heat and cover. Allow to sit an additional 2–3 minutes. Turn steak over and turn off heat. Allow to sit 4–6 minutes. Remove from heat and allow to rest. Carve and drizzle with olive oil and sprinkle with sea salt. Serve with lemon wedges.

Chef's Diet Options:
Try with well-trimmed leg of lamb, veal chops, or pork tenderloin.
Use your favorite herbs such as basil, thyme, savory, or even lavender.

Note: I like to serve flatiron steak with Tuscan Broccoli and Micro/baked Butternut Squash.

185

Flax-Crusted Pork Cutlet Piccata

Everyone learns how to make chicken or veal piccata in culinary school. It is a classic dish that is wonderful in its simplicity. Now that we are backing away from white flour, how are we going to replace dredging in flour, which is so important to this dish? Flaxseed is one good answer. The dish not only survives the change, but the flax adds a depth in flavor and "toastiness" that I think you will quite enjoy. I like to serve this with short-grained brown rice and my blanched greens combo. "Vive la différence!"

Makes 2 healthy portions

Ingredients:

2 (5- to 6-ounce) pork cutlets, pounded thin

4 cloves garlic, finely minced

2 sprigs thyme, stems removed

Salt and pepper to taste

⅓ cup ground flaxseed

2 tablespoons extra-virgin olive oil, plus additional for drizzling

1 tablespoon capers

Juice of 1 lemon

Directions:

Rub cutlets with the garlic and thyme and press them into the meat. Season with salt and pepper. Place flaxseed meal on a plate and place cutlets on top. Press the meal into the cutlets evenly.

Heat a nonstick pan over medium-high heat. Add the olive oil and swirl to coat the pan evenly. Add the cutlets and brown on first side (2–3 minutes), then turn over and brown the other side and cook through.

Remove the cutlets to warm plates. Quickly add the capers and lemon juice and a touch of olive oil. Pour equal amounts over the two cutlets. Serve with your favorite MyTendWell side dishes.

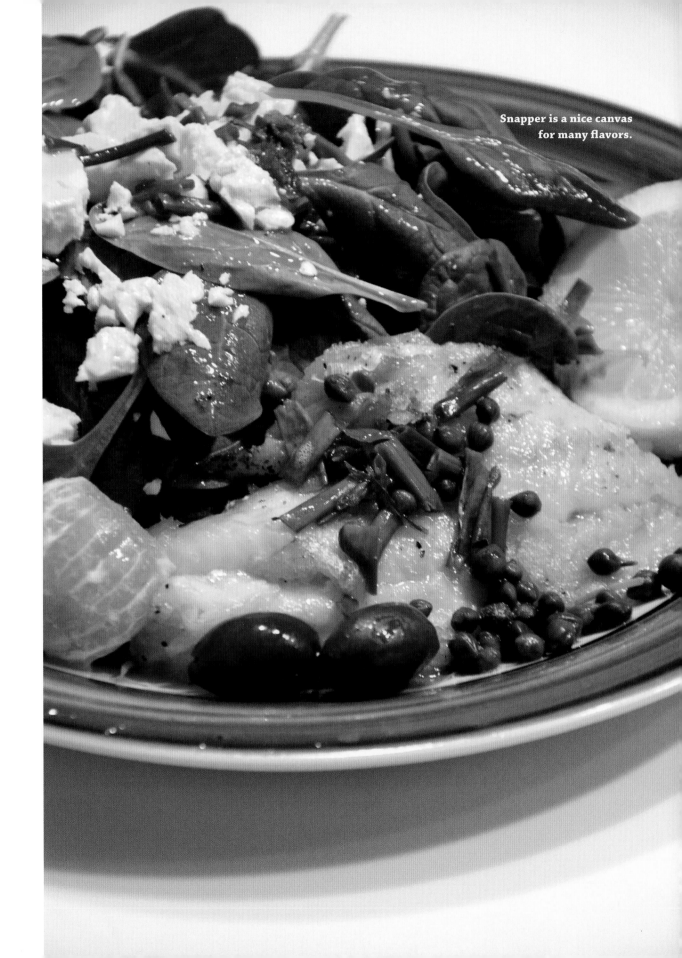

Snapper is a nice canvas
for many flavors.

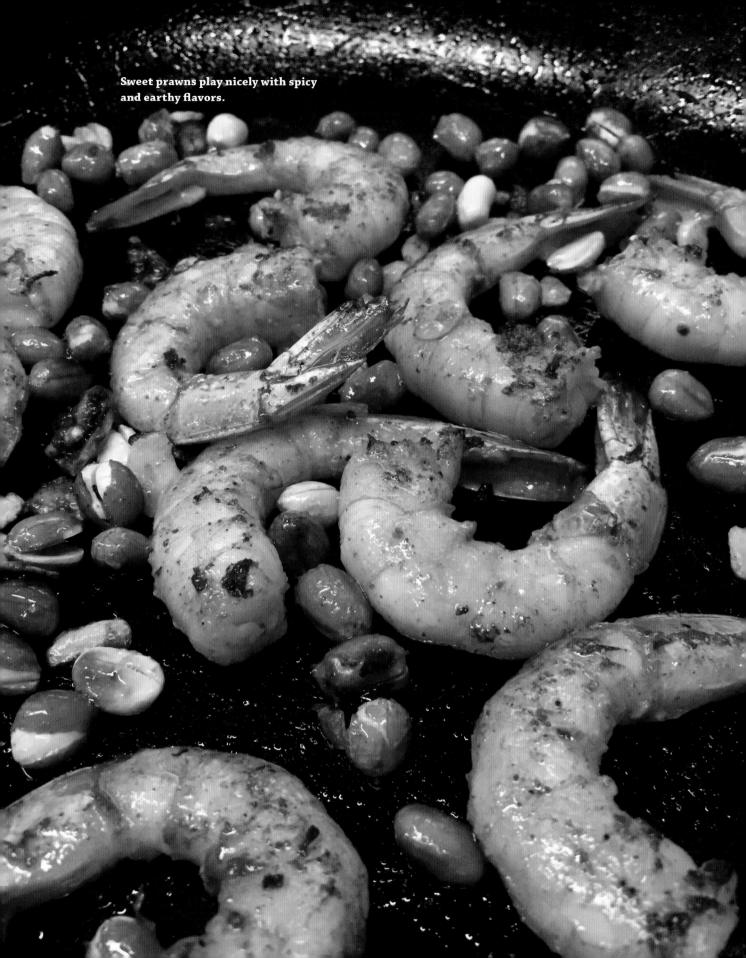

Sweet prawns play nicely with spicy and earthy flavors.

Pan-Roasted Prawns and Spinach with Peanuts

This is a great quick dish that you can make in minutes. I like to serve it with Ethiopian injera bread or brown rice. Top quality prawns are a key to taking this dish from GREAT to FANTASTIC. In Bloomington, we have a crew that brings us fresh seafood from the Gulf Coast once a month, and we line up to buy it. This seafood is soooo different from the frozen, imported, farmed stuff. Sweet and fatty with a touch of iodine—yum. Save the shells and make a nice broth. You can freeze the shells and make the stock later.

Makes 2 healthy servings

Ingredients:

10 large prawns, peeled and deveined

4 cloves garlic, minced

2 teaspoon Kitchen D'Orr Spice Blend (or
    1 teaspoon Chinese five-spice powder)

1 teaspoon cumin seeds

½ teaspoon cayenne pepper

2 teaspoons extra-virgin olive oil

½ cup raw peanuts

½ medium onion, finely chopped

½ red bell pepper, julienned

½ yellow bell pepper, julienned

1 6-ounce container baby spinach

Sea salt and freshly ground pepper to taste

1 lemon, cut in half

Hot sauce to accompany

Directions:

Place the prawns in a bowl with the garlic, spices, and oil. Toss and allow to marinate 10–15 minutes. Prepare your vegetables while shrimp is marinating.

Heat a 10-inch nonstick pan over high heat. Add prawns and marinade, allowing to color nicely on one side. Add peanuts and turn over prawns with tongs.

Quickly add onions and peppers, and stir-fry until peanuts are lightly browned. Quickly add spinach, turn off heat, and toss until spinach is wilted. Squeeze ½ lemon over the dish, season to taste with salt and pepper.

Serve on warm plates with remaining lemon, hot sauce, injera bread, or brown rice.

Roast Black Cod with Pancetta, Anise Seed, and Green Chickpeas

Always look for sustainable fish if available. Often this will be line-caught on smaller boats instead of caught in nets in large quantities. It is more expensive, but the price you pay is worth the small impact it has on the earth and the species. You can check online and find out the types of fish that are good for you and good for the ocean. The website seafood.edf.org is a good place to get the latest update. Black cod, or sablefish, is a rich and flavorful choice, but hake or haddock would also work in the preparation. As a reminder, animal and fish proteins should not be served in monumental portion sizes.

Makes 2 healthy servings

Ingredients:

1 pound of fish of choice (look for thick fillets)

2 teaspoons anise seeds

2 teaspoons garlic, minced

2 tablespoons extra-virgin olive oil—plus a little extra

1 tablespoon lemon juice or light vinegar

Sea salt and freshly ground pepper to taste

4 thin slices pancetta

2 cups frozen green Bengal chickpeas—may be found in West Indian markets (may use canned traditional chickpeas if unavailable)

1 cup tomato juice

Optional garnishes: Lemon or lime wedges, fresh cilantro, or chopped scallions

Directions:

Cut the fish into 4 equal portions and toss with the anise, garlic, olive oil, lemon juice, and salt and pepper. Place in fridge for 15–20 minutes.

Preheat the oven to 450 degrees.

Brush baking dish with a little olive oil. Place fish fillets in the dish and top each with a piece of pancetta. Pour over any remaining marinade. Toss the Bengal chickpeas in the tomato juice and pour around the fish.

Roast fish for 10–15 minutes or until the pancetta begins to crisp and the fish is just cooked through in the thickest part. Taste chickpeas and adjust seasoning with sea salt, freshly ground pepper, and lemon juice or vinegar. Serve with a wedge of lemon or lime.

West Indian Leg of Lamb with Mixed Herbs

Chef D cooks this dish when he is cooking for a crowd, often on Easter. But it doesn't have to be a holiday to celebrate this recipe; you can use it on lamb chops, saddle, or sirloin as well. This is a great marinade for lamb, goat, or other red meat, but it works equally well with poultry, pork, or even thick fish steaks. Marinate for 20 minutes to 24 hours depending on the thickness of the meat, then grill, roast, or put on the rotisserie. Cook with high heat until meat is nicely browned and crusty, and then turn the heat way down and cook to desired doneness. You could also make a full batch of the marinade, separate it out into small containers, and then refrigerate or freeze. You'll find it wonderful with different proteins and cooking methods.

Makes marinade for one leg of lamb, approximately 6–10 servings depending on size

Ingredients:

½ cup olive oil

5 key limes, thinly sliced

¼ cup brown cane sugar

1 bunch thyme, roughly chopped

1 bunch rosemary, roughly chopped

1 cup other herbs such as basil, chives, tarragon, mint, and/or scallions

2 heads garlic, roughly chopped

1 red onion, thinly sliced

1 tablespoon cracked black peppercorns

1 tablespoon crushed red pepper flakes

1 tablespoon cracked allspice berries

2 tablespoons Mellow Yellow Spice Blend or curry powder

1 tablespoon whole mustard seeds

4 bay leaves, crushed

1 tablespoon Thai bird peppers, dried

1 fresh red chili, roughly chopped

2 tablespoons fresh ginger, chopped

2 tablespoons sea salt

Directions:

Mix all ingredients for the marinade together in a glass or stainless steel bowl. Squeeze ingredients to encourage combination of flavors and release of juices.

For the lamb:

Break the lamb legs down into muscles. Remove most of the fat, leaving a thin protective cap. Your butcher should be able to do this, especially if you order it in advance. Reserve bones for soup stock. (If using poultry cut it into breasts, thighs, legs, and wings.)

Use enough marinade to give a good rub into the meat. Place the meat and a bit of extra marinade in ziplock bags, and squeeze out any air. Place in the refrigerator at least 2 hours or overnight.

Grill, roast, or bake to your taste. Red meats should be well caramelized on exterior and rosy inside and poultry cooked through.

Serve with tomato and cucumber salad.

Spaghetti Squash and Turkey and Quinoa Meatballs

I make the full batch of meatballs and use them throughout the week, but feel free to cut the ingredients in half if you want. They are good plain, with tomato sauce, in pita pockets, in minestrone or Italian wedding soup, or popped in the mouth cold as a high-protein snack!

Makes 4–6 healthy servings

Ingredients:

1 pound ground turkey

1 cup cooked quinoa

2 teaspoons granulated garlic

1 teaspoon ground cumin

½ teaspoon crushed red pepper flakes (or more to taste if you like spice)

1 teaspoon dried oregano

½ cup fresh herbs (mostly parsley mixed with scallions, basil, oregano, and/or other herbs you have on hand), chopped

Sea salt and freshly ground pepper to taste

2 ½ cups good chicken or turkey broth

1 cup homemade or favorite tomato sauce (look for one without sugar or corn syrup and thickeners, organic preferred)

1 medium spaghetti squash, cooked and prepared (see info below for cooking instructions)

Directions:

In a large bowl, combine the meat, quinoa, garlic, spices, and herbs, and season with salt and pepper. Make a mini meatball and microwave for 20 seconds or until cooked through. Taste and adjust seasoning. Roll into balls a bit smaller than golf balls.

In a 12- to 14-inch sauté pan with a cover, heat the broth and tomato sauce to a boil, and season to taste with salt, pepper, and chili flakes, if desired. Mix well and add the meatballs. Reduce heat to a simmer and cover with lid. Cook, simmering 25–30 minutes, until balls reach 160 degrees in the center. Remove from heat and allow to cool in sauce.

Place in storage containers and put equal amounts of cooking liquid in each container. Cool to room temperature and refrigerate or freeze until needed.

To serve, heat meatballs with sauce and spaghetti squash. Make a nice pile of squash in center of warm plate, spoon three meatballs and sauce around. Drizzle with a little of your best quality extra-virgin olive oil. Accompany with some grated cheese if you like, your favorite salad, and your best whole-grain baguette.

Note on cooking spaghetti squash:

Spaghetti squash is great for replacing empty carbs from white pasta with something nutritious. Don't get me wrong, I'm not a hater. Pasta, especially whole grain varieties, is part of the joy of life. It just can't be a daily crutch. Cooked spaghetti squash will last 5–7 days in the fridge, but I doubt it will, because I know you'll eat it all up. You can use it for all sorts of things: omelets in the morning, a salad or sandwich stuffer at lunch, or a vegetable side dish at dinner. Like pasta, it takes on the flavors you add to it.

No recipe needed: This is very easy and I usually do it in the microwave at home. Carefully cut the squash in half lengthwise and scoop out the seeds (these are great to pan roast for a crispy snack or salad topper). Place cut side down in a Pyrex or microwavable ceramic dish. Add about ¼ inch of water. Cover with cling film and microwave on high heat for 6–10 minutes depending on size. When done you should be able to take a fork and rake it crossways from surface to skin removing crisp/tender strands of "spaghetti." Do not overcook! It is better to undercook and put back in for a few minutes than to turn it into mush. Cool to room temperature. Refrigerate until needed, up to 5 days.

To cook pumpkin or squash seeds:

Place the seeds and squash membrane in a bowl of room-temperature water. Take your fingers and mix them around well until the seeds separate from the membrane. Carefully skim the seeds off the top of the water and put on a paper towel. Go through remaining membrane and retrieve remaining seeds.

Place seeds in an appropriate-sized nonstick sauté pan and add ¼ cup water and a pinch of salt. Cook over medium heat, stirring occasionally until water evaporates. Add a drizzle of olive oil, granulated garlic, and freshly ground pepper. Cook, stirring occasionally on medium-low heat until crisp. You can also do larger batches in a medium-hot oven. Cool to room temperature. Store lightly covered until ready to use . . . if they last that long.

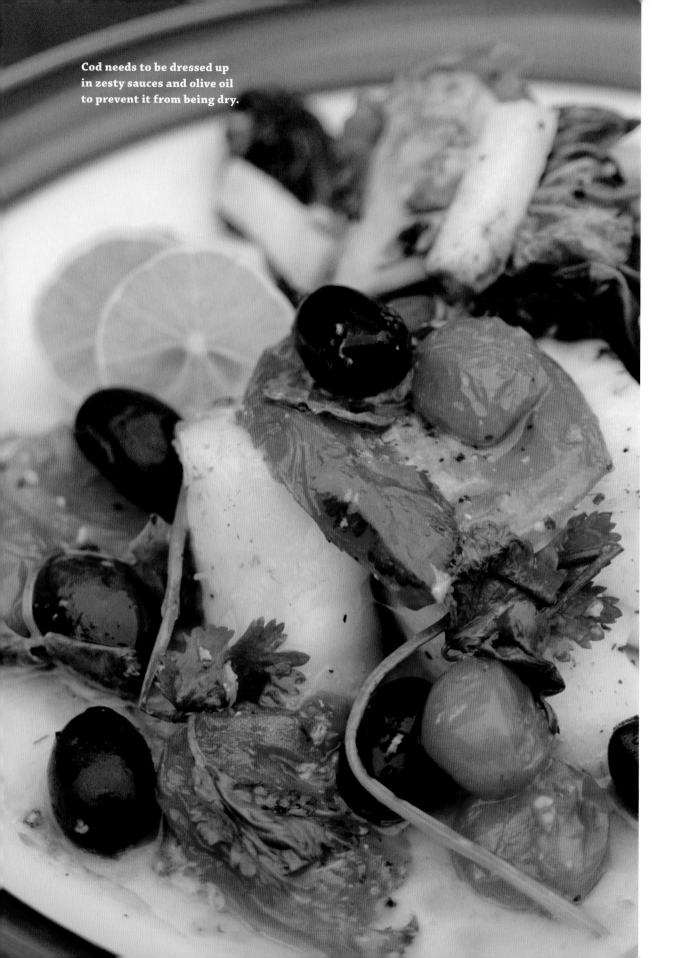

Cod needs to be dressed up
in zesty sauces and olive oil
to prevent it from being dry.

Spelt Pasta with Rainbow Chard, Tomatoes, and Garlic

Many people who go on a diet never think of going to a health food store, but if you are dieting to become healthy, not just beautiful, a health food store is the place you should go first. One thing you will find there is wonderful whole wheat, spelt, and sprouted-grain pastas. Give them a try. They are more toothsome and deeper in flavor but can be tricky to prepare. Make sure you read the label and follow instructions. Because of the lack of strong gluten and eggs in many of these pastas, they cook rapidly and often are best if quickly rinsed under cold water after draining.

This is a great lunch or satisfying early dinner when you need a long-term energy boost.

Makes 4 healthy servings

Ingredients:

½ pound spelt, whole wheat, or sprouted-grain penne (try Food for Life, Ezekiel 4:9 brand)

2 tablespoons olive oil

4 cloves garlic, minced

1 large bunch rainbow chard (or kale or beet greens or other sturdy green), roughly chopped

¼ teaspoon ground nutmeg

Salt and pepper to taste

1 large beefsteak tomato, cut medium dice

2 tablespoons extra-virgin olive oil

3 tablespoons Parmesan cheese, grated

Directions:

Cook pasta according to directions in a medium saucepan. Drain and rinse pasta quickly under cold water to stop the cooking.

Return empty pan to the heat and add olive oil. When hot, add garlic and sauté until lightly golden with a nutty aroma. Quickly add the greens and stir to incorporate the garlic so it doesn't burn.

Once greens have wilted, season with nutmeg, salt, and pepper. Add the tomato and return the drained pasta to the pot. Heat pasta through while lightly tossing and remove from heat. Finish pasta with the extra-virgin olive oil and cheese. Taste and adjust seasoning as needed with salt and pepper.

Chef's Diet Options:
Add a little lemon zest.
Add diced firm tofu or low-fat feta.
Add olives or capers.
Add nuts.
Replace greens with green beans or broccoli.
Add a handful of chopped basil, mint, or cilantro.

TO SWEET OR NOT TO SWEET

To sweets or not to sweet . . . that is the question?

The MyTendWell Lifestyle Plan philosophy is *everything in moderation*. You can't start another program, you have to start a new lifestyle. You will slip, but you don't have to fall. If you fall, get right back up . . . unless there is a slice of chocolate cake down there.

But seriously, ladies and germs . . . you can't say you'll never have ice cream again, or cakes, or pies, or tarts, or puddings, or candy, or cookies, or brownies—well, you get the picture. What we do suggest is that you cut the cravings with whole fresh fruits, nice cups of herbal tea, a few nuts, a square of dark chocolate, a handful of homemade granola, a dried fig, or a piece of low-fat string cheese. And don't forget lots of water! Add a little lemon juice or cider vinegar to the water, and you'll slow down and realize you are on your way to a binge.

However, we did want to offer a few recipes that you can make to satisfy that sweet tooth without getting yourself in too much trouble. These cut the evil empire's control but still allow you to celebrate life. They mostly are high in fiber, which fills your gut and reduces your hunger.

The longer you resist your temptations, the less often they will occur. If you are able to stay away from the evil empire long enough, you will actually find that your old "friends" won't taste as good as they used to. If you cut artificial or highly sweetened "products" out of your life, the "real food" you are now eating will be what you want to binge on.

Quick sorbets and frozen yogurts are simple and satisfying. Just place 3 cups of your favorite frozen fruit (avoiding seedy berries) with 1 cup of low-fat yogurt and ¼ cup of your favorite sweetener like agave, maple syrup, or honey. Add a touch of lemon or lime juice for a little zing and blend until smooth in a blender or food processor. Pour into freezer containers and freeze for 20–30 minutes and you're set!

We all remember our elementary school cafeteria line "fruit cocktail." It wasn't that special. But with the wide variety of fresh produce available at farmers' markets and at the grocery store, fruit salad is something to celebrate.

Fruit salad is a great dessert and you can vary it with what is in season or by color. I love tossing all green fruits like grapes, kiwi, honeydew, green apples, and some mint together and make a "Green Goddess Salad!" Try this with all red, purple, or orange fruit. They make striking presentations. Fruit skewers are also a fun way to get people to eat more fruit. Try making "Pride Day" rainbow brochettes by sticking a variety of colorful fruit and berries on a skewer and serve with a maple and yogurt dip.

Frozen Grape Sorbet Bombs

Nothing could be easier than this! Chef D is a late-night snacker and when he is jonesing for a sweet treat, this is his healthy go-to option. For the most nutritious option, choose seedless grapes with the darkest red or purple skins. They have the most phytonutrients. We suggest you always have these in your freezer in case of an unexpected snack attack! You can also eat other frozen fruits like blueberries and peaches, but you may have to use a spoon for those, whereas the grapes are in their own little serving packages. For fruits that contain more water and freeze harder, you may have to allow them to sit at room temperature for 10–15 minutes to soften. For a plated dessert, try layering frozen fruit, yogurt, and agave in a glass bowl or shallow cup.

Ingredients:

1 pound seedless grapes—choose several varieties for a more colorful dessert.

Directions:

Wash grape bunches well and put them in a ziplock bag. Freeze overnight. With scissors, cut off the amount you want to eat and return remaining grapes to the freezer. Enjoy!

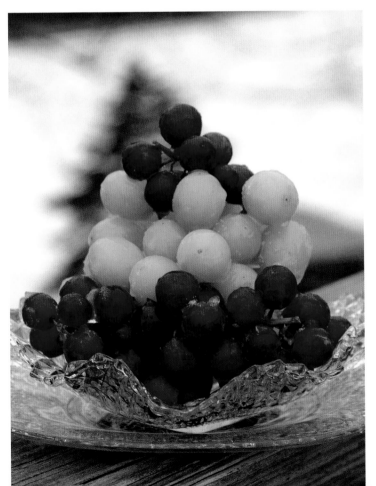

Frozen grapes.

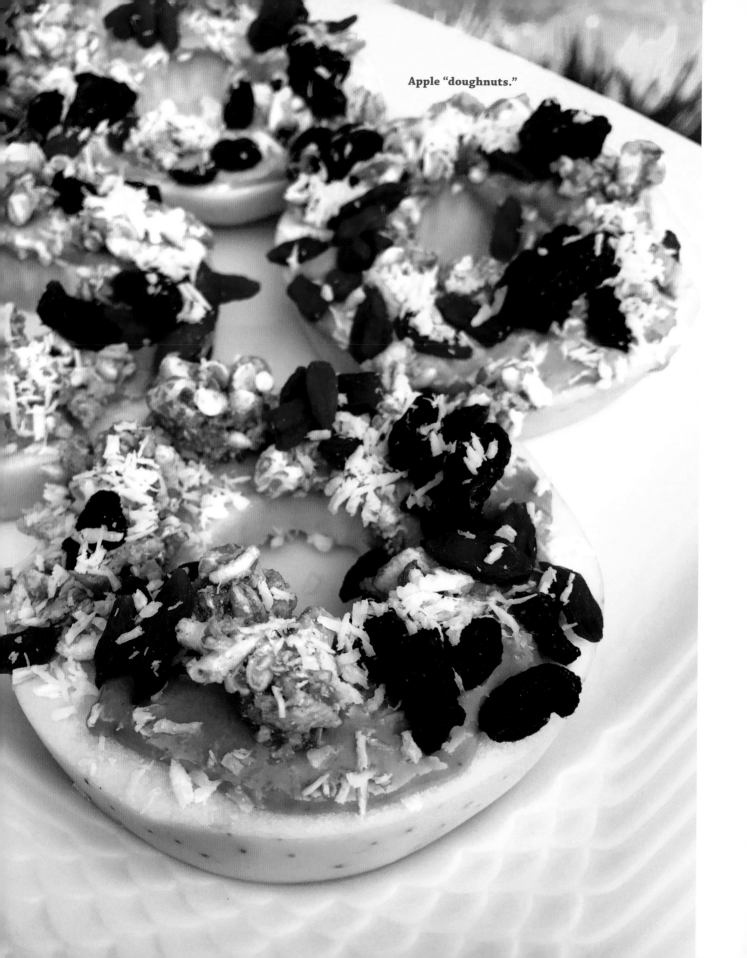

Apple "doughnuts."

Apple "Doughnuts" with Nut Butter and Coconut

This is a simple dessert, but one that satisfies. It also makes a great midmorning or afternoon snack. You can top them with any type of nut butter and then use your healthy pantry to choose your toppings. You can even make it a DIY dessert by placing small bowls of ingredients on a tray and having fellow diners pick their favorite combinations.

Note: If you want to cut your apples more than 15–20 minutes in advance, brush the cut sides with a little honey thinned with lemon juice to prevent them from browning.

Makes 4–5 healthy doughnuts

Ingredients:

1 large apple

½ cup cashew or favorite nut butter

½ cup favorite granola or whole grain cereal, such as Kashi GoLean

½ cup dried fruit, such as raisins, goji berries, chopped apricots

½ cup shredded sugar-free coconut

Directions:

Cut apple into 4–5 thick rounds. Using a small round or crimpled biscuit cutter, cut and compost the star-like center core. Top apple ring with nut butter and sprinkle with cereal, fruit, and coconut. Serve quickly.

Blender Banana Frozen Yogurt

Bananas have a nice balance of richness, sweetness, and creaminess. They are also economical and full of potassium. Chef D likes to buy the ones on sale that already are spotted and turning soft; then he takes them home, peels them, and puts them in the freezer for later use in smoothies and desserts. Try adding some cinnamon or cardamom to your mix to make something a little more exotic.

Note: You can also take these frozen bananas, cut into bite-sized pieces, and dip them in dark chocolate for banana sushi bites.

Ingredients:

3 frozen bananas, cut into small rounds

1 cup low-fat yogurt

¼ cup maple syrup (or honey or agave)

Juice of 1 lime plus 1 teaspoon zest (or ½ lemon and zest)

¼ teaspoon cinnamon or a few cardamom seeds (removed from the pods)

Directions:

Combine all ingredients in the bowl of your blender or food processor and process until very smooth and creamy. Put mixture into a chilled freezer container and place it in the deep freeze for 2–3 hours or overnight, until it is firm but not hard. If the "ice cream" gets too hard, just pull it out of the freezer 10–15 minutes before serving to soften.

Note: Try garnishing with a dollop of yogurt, chopped dark chocolate, and nuts.

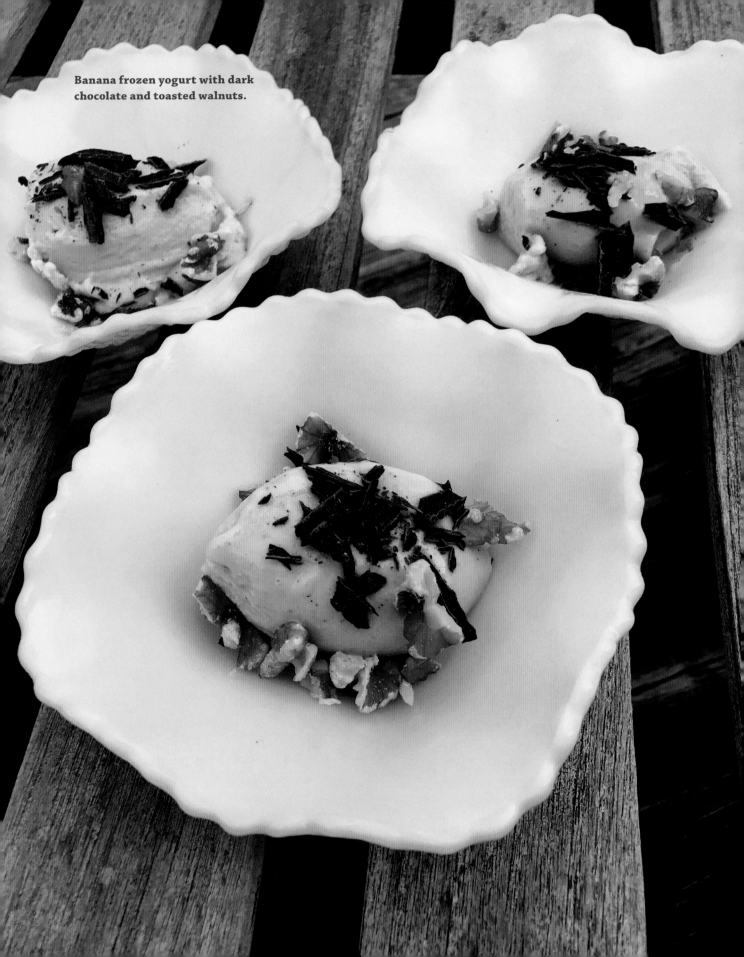

Banana frozen yogurt with dark chocolate and toasted walnuts.

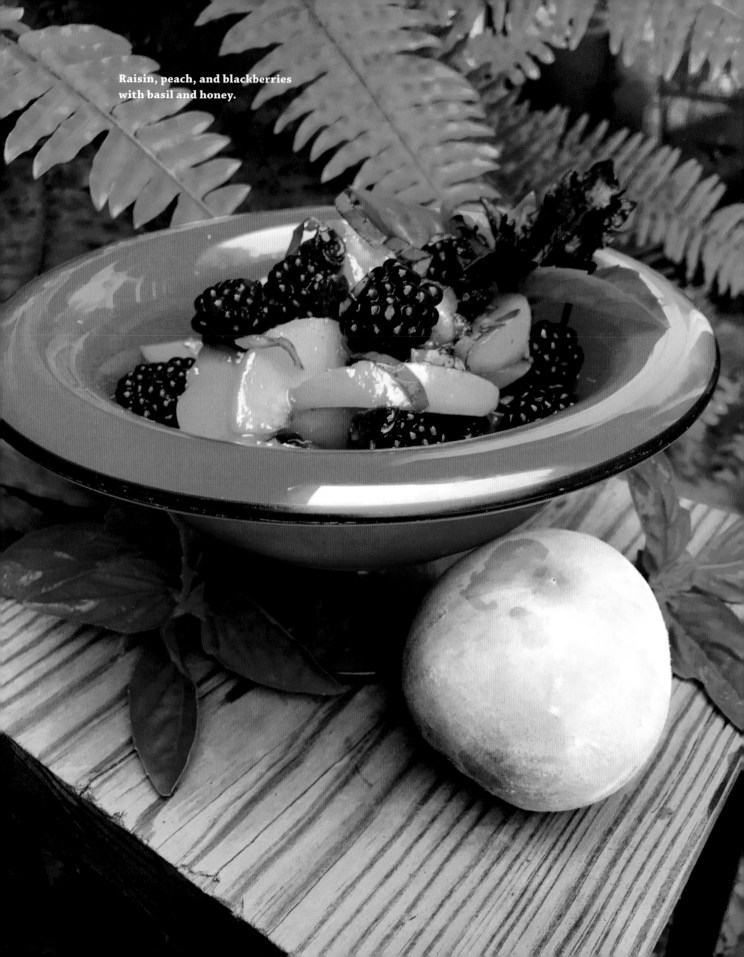

Raisin, peach, and blackberries
with basil and honey.

Peach, Raisin, and Blackberry Compote with Spices, Basil, and Honey

This is a great recipe to make and keep in the fridge. It is good not just as a dessert but also as a snack or even a breakfast with some whole grain cereal. It couldn't be easier to make and can be served on its own or with nuts over yogurt as a parfait. We also like it as an accompaniment to some aged cheddar, blue, or other sharp cheese.

This sweet will give you a "happy mouth!" This recipe is designed to be chewed! The different textures of the fresh and dried fruit, the crunch of the lemon zest, the explosive flavor from the chiffonade of basil, and the haunting warmth of the cayenne and cinnamon make it memorable.

Note: Peaches are one of the few fruits that you can usually count on being good frozen, but they can be hit-or-miss fresh. There is nothing more wonderful than a perfect peach or more disappointing than a bad one. Problem is, they can look exactly the same. The issue is the way they are picked and stored. Peaches picked underripe and refrigerated can be bland and mealy.

Makes 4–6 healthy servings

Ingredients:

3 cups sliced peaches, frozen

½ cup raisins

3 tablespoons organic honey

Juice and zest of ½ organic lemon

½ teaspoon cinnamon

1 knife's point cayenne pepper or to taste (optional)

½ pint blackberries

3–4 basil leaves, cut into thin ribbons

Directions:

Thaw peaches overnight in the refrigerator or microwave for 3–4 minutes in a glass bowl. Add raisins, honey, citrus, and spices and allow to sit at room temperature until the raisins absorb the excess juices, about 1–2 hours. Refrigerate until well chilled and add blackberries and basil just before serving.

Pineapple Pizzas with Berries, Raspberry and Cardamom "Marinara," and Coconut "Mozzarella"

This is a pretty dessert that is all about the ingredients. If the pineapple isn't really ripe, the center core will be tough and fibrous. To pick a good pineapple, look for one that is turning golden, smells fragrant, and is softening but not mushy; also, the green crown should be starting to turn brown at the tips, and, when tugged, a leaf will detach without too much trouble. Try topping with other items such as yogurt, dried fruit, and toasted nuts.

Makes 4 healthy servings

Ingredients:

1 cup fresh or frozen raspberries (thawed)

1 tablespoon honey (or agave or maple)

Seeds from one cardamom pod

½–¾ of a ripe pineapple, top and bottom removed, peeled, sliced into ½-inch thick rounds

4 strawberries, washed and diced

½ cup blueberries

8–10 blackberries, cut in half

¼ cup sugar-free shredded organic coconut

Directions:

For the marinara, combine the raspberries, sweetener, and cardamom seeds in a blender and puree until smooth. Chill until needed.

Just before serving, place a pineapple round on each plate. Spoon over a little of the marinara in the middle of the pineapple. Decorate with berries and sprinkle with shredded coconut "mozzarella." Garnish with pineapple leaves.

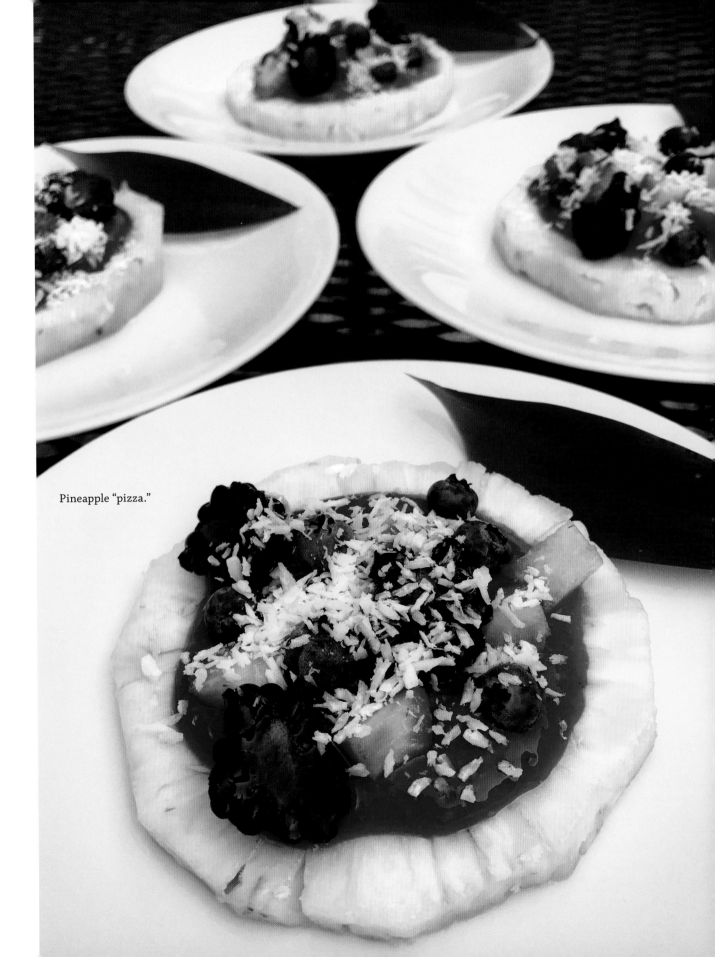

Pineapple "pizza."

Strawberries with agave.

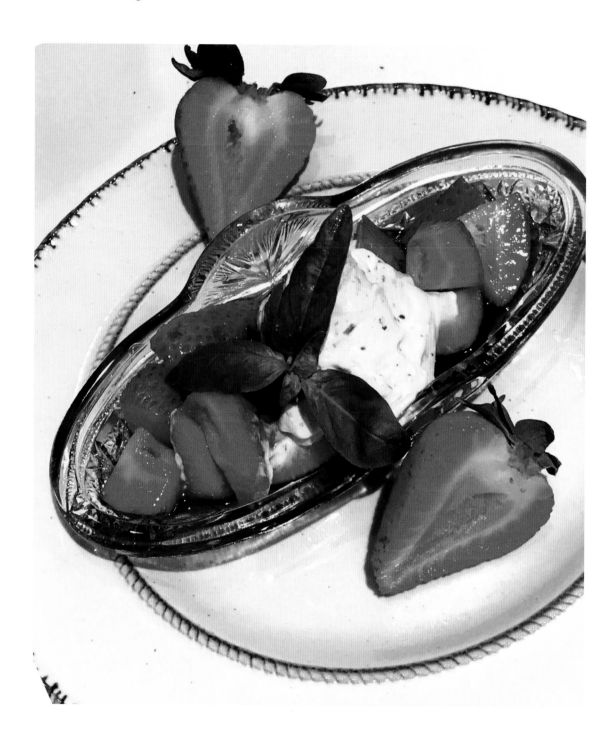

Key Lime Vinegar Dipping Sauce

This is a great thin dipping sauce for raw or cooked seafood—light and refreshing but spicy and lasting. It's also nice for dipping Asian summer rolls. I even use it as a marinade for rich salmon and other items for the grill.

Makes ¾ cup

Ingredients:

½ cup white vinegar

Juice of 3 key limes

1 tablespoon Thai fish sauce

3 cloves garlic, thinly sliced

½ teaspoon cracked black pepper

2 tablespoons honey or agave

Chilies to taste (I use Thai bird peppers)

Optional: Minced ginger and/or fresh cilantro, mint, or scallions as needed

Directions:

Mix all the ingredients together and adjust seasoning to your own taste.

Powerhouse Peppermint Pesto

During mint season, make a big batch of this to freeze for wintertime enjoyment. This recipe may be quartered or halved if desired. It's great to share with family and friends. Use on whole grain tabbouleh, couscous salad, grilled eggplant or other veggies, meats, poultry, or seafood. Also, it makes a great spread for sandwiches or pita pockets. It's perfect for lamb!

Makes 1 quart

Ingredients:

5 cups parsley, chopped

8 cups peppermint leaves

1 jalapeño, roughly chopped

10 cloves garlic, crushed

2 cups extra-virgin olive oil (for flavor and health benefits)

2 cups olive oil (for volume)

Salt and pepper to taste

Optional: 1 cup lightly roasted almonds

Directions:

In food processor, process parsley, mint, jalapeño, and garlic until fairly smooth. Add almonds, if desired, and pulse until they are approximately quartered. Slowly add oils until emulsified. Season to taste. Freeze in small containers. Serve at room temperature.

Island Curry Vinaigrette

We use this dressing on our Caribbean slaw at the restaurant, but it is also great on a variety of salads or with poached or grilled shrimp and other seafood.

Makes 2 cups

Ingredients:

2 tablespoons extra-virgin olive oil

¼ cup shallots, chopped

½ tablespoon garlic, finely chopped

2 tablespoons curry powder

½ tablespoon turmeric

¼ cup cider vinegar

1 tablespoon honey

1 cup vegetable oil

Juice of 2 lemons plus zest of ½ a lemon

½ tablespoon salt

1 teaspoon pepper

Favorite hot sauce

Directions:

Heat the olive oil in a heavy-bottomed saucepan and add the shallots and garlic. Cook slowly until transparent but uncolored. Add curry and turmeric and continue to cook to bring the flavors together. Deglaze with cider vinegar and place in a blender. Add honey and vegetable oil and blend until smooth. Add lemon juice and zest, and season with salt, pepper, and hot sauce to taste. Store in refrigerator for up to 7 days.

Miso Blender Dressing

This is a great everyday vinaigrette. Use on salads and slaws of all types. Also makes a great dip for veggies and other snacks. Keeps in the fridge for 5–7 days.

Makes 1 cup

Ingredients:

¼ cup brown miso (available at Japanese markets and health food stores)

¼ cup water

2 tablespoons Chinese black vinegar (or balsamic)

Juice of 1 lemon

1 clove garlic

½ tablespoon fresh ginger, minced

1 tablespoon fresh jalapeño, seeds removed, minced

½ cup olive oil

2 tablespoons toasted sesame oil (available in the international aisle of most supermarkets)

Salt and pepper to taste

Directions:

Combine the miso, water, vinegar, lemon juice, garlic, ginger, and jalapeño in a blender and pulse to combine. While running, drizzle in the olive and sesame oils. Thin as needed with extra water. Season to taste. Be careful with the salt, as the miso and black vinegar are already very salty.

Lemon and Spice Tahini Dressing (a.k.a. Tahini Mayo)

Love this stuff on most anything. It adds richness and depth of flavor to sandwiches, salads, crudités, hot or cold brown rice or grains, or grilled or chilled poultry or fish. Keep some around at all times.

Note: I like to make mine thick, close to a mayonnaise. That way I can use it for a dip or sandwich spread, or I can thin it as needed for a salad or sauce.

Makes 2 cups

Ingredients:

⅓ cup sesame tahini (ground sesame paste)

3 cloves garlic, roughly chopped

1 teaspoon ground cumin

½ teaspoon ground cardamom

½ teaspoon cayenne

1 teaspoon sea salt

2 lemons, zest of one, juice of both

¼ cup good quality olive oil

1 cup water

Additional sea salt and freshly ground pepper to taste

Optional: ¼ cup herbs (mostly parsley but add cilantro, chives, mint, etc.), chopped

Optional: Your favorite hot sauce

Directions:

Place all ingredients in food processor or blender and pulse until dressing comes together. Add additional water if needed. Season to your taste with salt and pepper, citrus, herbs, and hot sauce.

Tofu Rouille

The forefather of this recipe comes from sunny coastal Provence. My recipe cuts the fat, but keeps the saffron, garlic, and spices. Refrigerate leftover rouille to use with grilled meats, fish, sandwiches, baked potatoes, and steamed broccoli and cauliflower. The sauce is great with crudités or thinned with a touch of vinegar and used as a salad dressing.

Makes 2 ½ cups

Ingredients:

1 potato, peeled and roughly diced

¼ cup water

1 teaspoon saffron threads

2 cloves garlic, peeled and roughly chopped

1 ½ teaspoons chili powder

¾ pound firm tofu, drained and lightly pressed to remove excess water

¼ cup extra-virgin olive oil

10 drops Tabasco

Salt and freshly ground pepper

Directions:

Cook the potato in boiling water until tender, drain and place in a bowl. Lightly mash the potato with a fork and allow the steam to escape.

In a small saucepan, bring water to a boil. Add the saffron, remove the pan from the heat, and steep the saffron for 8–10 minutes. Combine the potato, saffron liquid, garlic, chili powder, tofu, and oil in a blender or food processor, and puree until the mixture is smooth. Season with the Tabasco, salt, and pepper to taste.

ROUILLE

Rouille is the rusty, sunny-colored mayonnaise-like sauce from the south of France. It is garlicky and has a slight punch of chilies. Classically served with bouillabaisse, I like it as a sandwich spread, vegetable dip, or garnishing sauce.

Tomato and Caper Vinaigrette

This vinaigrette is great with all fish and chicken that has been grilled, poached, or roasted.

Note: Additional chopped herbs such as tarragon, basil, or chives may be added to taste just before serving. If added too far in advance, they will discolor.

Makes 1 cup

Ingredients:

½ cup tomato concasse (ripe tomatoes, peeled, seeded, and roughly chopped)

Juice of 2 lemons

1 teaspoon garlic, chopped

2 tablespoons Spanish Xeres (sherry) vinegar

4 tablespoons extra-virgin olive oil (top quality)

1 teaspoon Brittany sea salt

1 ½ tablespoons capers

1 teaspoon lemon zest, brunoise

Pepper to taste

Directions:

In a blender, combine the tomato, lemon juice, garlic, vinegar, olive oil, and sea salt and puree until combined but still slightly chunky. Pour into a storage container and add the capers and lemon zest brunoise. Season to taste.

JUST AROUND THE CORNER . . .

Wellness is an integration of all that life is . . . family, work, food, play, loss, laughter. Moving toward optimal wellness is a lifelong pursuit that requires continued learning and dedication to ourselves. Learn more in the next *MyTendWell* book!

And don't forget, drive by . . . don't drive through.

Love you and see you soon!

Chef D and Dr. K

Happy Cooking

DANIEL

Keep Moving

Dr. K

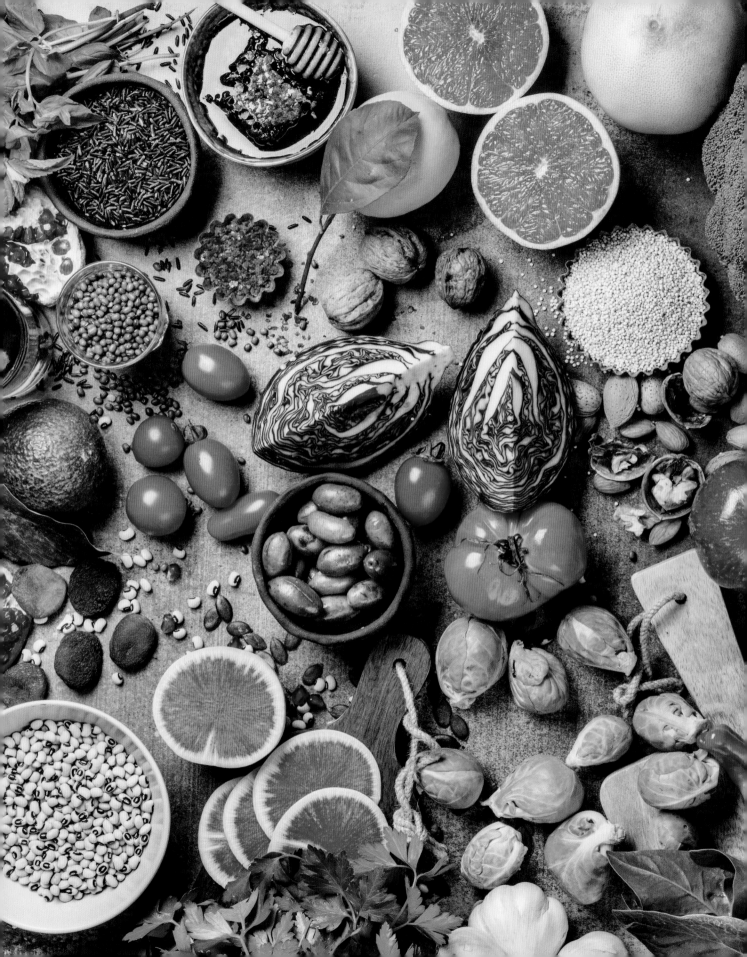

HEALTHY FOODS GLOSSARY

alliums in the family: Alliums are extremely important in cooking. They offer a wide variety of flavors depending on variety, length of cooking, and cooking method. The allium family contains all the oniony and garlicky flavored plants, both wild and cultivated. They range from chives, scallions, garlic, and shallots to the larger white, Spanish, and red onion bulbs. All can be enjoyed raw for their aggressive biting flavor, but cooking often brings out a softer side of the alliums' personality. Herbalists often use garlic against infection, as a blood-clotting deterrent, and to lower blood pressure. It also keeps vampires away as well as unwanted suitors: that would be anyone who doesn't like garlic IS an unwanted suitor.

amaranth: Amaranth is a whole grain that is actually a seed that has been used for at least 8,000 years. The Aztecs relied on the seed as a staple of their diet. The Spanish tried to defeat the indigenous people by destroying the plant, but, luckily for us, the seeds turned out to be even more defiant than the people. It is gluten-free and a great source of all the essential amino acids, including lysine, which is lacking in most grains. High in fiber and a good source of magnesium and iron, amaranth is a fabulous addition to your diet. Amaranth has an earthy, nutty flavor that is great in breads, makes a unique breakfast cereal, and becomes a polenta-like porridge.

animal protein: Classically, in human history, animal proteins delivered all the essential amino acids we needed from food. Other protein-rich foods like fruits, veggies, grains, seeds, and nuts are missing one or more of these essential amino acids. Proper food combinations will easily give you all the proteins you need, but accomplishing this is an important task. A meal plan containing too much animal protein can result in chronic diseases such as cardiovascular issues, diabetes, cancer, osteoporosis, and weight issues.

apples: Apples are full of a fiber called pectin. A medium-sized apple contains about 4 grams of fiber. Pectin is classed as a soluble, fermentable, and viscous fiber, a combination that gives it a huge list of health benefits: whiter teeth, fighter of Alzheimer's and Parkinson's diseases, cancer, and diabetes. Apples may also prevent diarrhea and constipation or help you through it.

artichokes: A true superfood, artichokes are low in calories and fat and high in fiber. Artichokes aid in the overall reduction in total cholesterol, are an excellent source of vitamins, folic acid, silymarin, caffeic acid, and ferulic acid. They are rich in minerals like copper, calcium, potassium, iron, manganese, and phosphorus, as well as potassium, an important component of cell and body fluids, which helps control heart rate and blood pressure by countering the effects of sodium. The first time my mom cooked artichokes, we ended up going out for dinner. But sixty years later, she's a pro!

asparagus: In ancient times it was thought to be an aphrodisiac, and now we know it does have some wonderful nutrients that stimulate our bodies. Asparagus spears come in several colors and sizes from purple, to green, to white. It is a member of the lily family of plants and is best locally grown in the spring. Asparagus is high in vitamin K and foliate and contains the amino acid asparagines, a detoxifying compound that can help destroy carcinogens. It is anti-inflammatory, helps regulate blood sugar, and has a wide variety of antioxidants. Great hot or cold!

avocado: One of my favorite fruits, avocados are full of healthy fats and can bring richness to any meal from breakfast to a late-night snack. There are many types of avocados throughout the world in many different colors, shapes, and sizes. One variety can reach up to 3 pounds. Haas avocados are the most popular in the United States. Avocados do not contain any cholesterol or *sodium* and are low in *saturated fat*.

baba ghanoush (eggplant and tahini dip): In Arabic, *baba* means father and *ghanoush* means spoiled. This is a dish that is so good that you can serve it on Father's Day for that spoiled vegetarian dad in your life.

barley: This is a wonderful grain to have in your pantry. Barley can replace rice in many dishes such as soups, salads, and side dishes. Pearled barley is the most readily available type in the market. "Pearled" means that the barley has been hulled, but also polished, removing much of the bran, making it much faster to cook but also a little less nutritious. One of my favorite salads is cooked and chilled barley, tossed with cucumbers, mint, cherry tomatoes, and sesame vinaigrette.

basil: Everyone loves basil, but fewer know how good it is for you. It is known to have anti-inflammatory and antibacterial properties. Vitamin K in basil is essential for production of clotting factors in the blood and plays a vital role in bone strengthening and mineralization. Basil herb contains a good amount of minerals like potassium, manganese, copper, and magnesium and its leaves are an excellent source of iron. Toss whole leaves in your salad bowl and put them on sandwiches and in wraps. Basil is great in breakfast egg dishes as well.

beans (fresh, dried, canned, or refried): Beans, beans, the magical fruit . . . that can lower cholesterol! Beans are a great source of fiber and protein, making them a staple of many diets around the world. Beans are thought to fight cancer, lower cholesterol, aid in weight loss, and help in managing diabetes. But beans may cause migraines, increase gout issues, and raise blood pressure when combined with some medications, for some people. They can also interfere with vitamin absorption, so make sure you eat plenty of leafy greens with your beans. And last, they can cause flatulence, so it is a good idea to cook them with fennel, caraway, lemon balm, and other herbs. Also, change your soaking water and discard it before cooking, and rinse all canned legumes. Another way thought to reduce gassiness is to cook legumes with acidic foods containing citrus or vinegar.

bee pollen: This is a "new age" ingredient that has been around for thousands of years. I know that I have felt better when taking it, and I love my bees . . . especially the queens! It has been claimed to *bee* an energy enhancer, lung tonic, skin soother, immune system waker-upper, and even an allergy preventer, but . . . ? I thought pollen was what caused allergies? I do know beekeepers who swear by it. They say they have fewer allergies when keeping bees and do enjoy a spoon of bee pollen with some fresh fruit or dairy protein to start the day.

(bodacious) berries: Blackberries, strawberries, blueberries, raspberries, gooseberries, currants, loganberries, cranberries, boysenberries, strawberries, and cranberries are big on antioxidants. These seem to help the body fight oxidative stress caused by free radicals that can lead to illness. If you can't find fresh berries, frozen (unsweetened) berries are a good substitute.

black pepper: As far as I'm concerned, one can't find much wrong with the black peppercorn, except the occasional sneeze. Black, white, and green peppercorns come from the *Piperaceae* family of plant. It is native to Kerala, the southern state of ***India***, but is grown throughout the tropical world. Brazil is now one of the largest producers. Black peppercorns are picked underdeveloped and allowed to dry, creating a wonderfully floral note. White peppercorns are fully developed and harder, they are also more "hot" to my taste. Green peppercorns are picked green and pickled or dehydrated; they are less spicy than either black or white and can be eaten whole in sauces and other preparations. (Pink peppercorns are not truly pepper but a dried fragrant berry from another species of plant.) Pepper has long been used by humans as a cooking ingredient and a medicine. It is thought to aid in issues including respiratory disorders, coughs, the common cold, ***constipation***, indigestion, ***anemia***, impotency, muscular strains, dental disease, pyorrhea, ***diarrhea***, and ***heart*** disease.

brunoise: This is a term used in French cooking meaning items diced in very small cubes. *Brunoise* adds color, flavor, and texture to all kinds of recipes and sauces.

buckwheat: Although wheat is in its name, there is no gluten in buckwheat. Buckwheat is not a grass-like wheat and is more closely related to rhubarb, sorrel, and knotweed. Its seeds may be cooked whole or ground into flour and used in a wide variety of recipes. I love the buckwheat crepes, served in Brittany, France, and traditional Japanese buckwheat noodles served in a chilled broth with egg yolk. This ingredient is a powerhouse of fiber and an antioxidant flavonoid called rutin, which regulates fluid retention and helps maintain a healthy digestive system.

Buckwheat is a gift for the heart, helping to reduce bad cholesterol. As for folks who are dieting, buckwheat should be your best friend. It has tons of fiber and protein, so it keeps you feeling full and energetic. It helps control your electrolyte levels, blood pressure, and the balance of your sugar levels. Ground buckwheat flour should be stored in your refrigerator to prevent it from becoming rancid; the whole kernels can be stored in an airtight container in a cool, dark place.

bulgur (toasted cracked wheat): This grain has been used for hundreds of years in Armenia, Syria, Israel, Palestine, and Turkey but is also used extensively in Indian cuisine. It is most famous in the States when tossed with tomatoes, parsley, and cucumbers as the main ingredient in tabbouleh. But bulgur is much more than a one hit wonder, it is also brilliant in pilafs, soups, stuffings, and baked goods. I even like to make vegetarian chili and Bolognese by allowing it to stand in for ground beef.

callaloo: I lived in the Caribbean for two years and loved every minute of it: the sun, the food, the beaches, and, most of all, the people. The people of the islands sustain themselves on "provisions." Those are the daily roots, wild herbs, greens, and fruits that can basically be found no matter how rich or how poor you are. Callaloo is basically the "wild spinach" that is most available on whichever island you find yourself hungry on. It might be the greens of the taro root on one island (which must be cooked) or the leaf of a wild amaranth plant on another. Many island dishes like Jamaican "run down" and Anguillan stew use their callaloo to feed the soul of the island. "Ya Mon, it's Irie."

cashews: The cashew tree is native to Brazil. When I am in Brazil I love drinking fresh cashew smoothies at the juice stand. The cashew nut is actually the seed of this fruit that hangs in a shell below the succulent soft fruit. Cashews are rich in iron, phosphorus, selenium, magnesium, and zinc. They are also a good source of phytochemicals, antioxidants, and protein. Try using cashews to make cashew milk and cashew flour. The copper in them helps to eliminate free radicals, and, although they taste rich, they have a lower fat content than many other nuts. They are said to calm the nerves and prevent gallstones. People who have small snacks of nuts seem to do better maintaining a healthy diet than others who hit the doNUT shop.

cheese (my greatest weakness): Americans eat between 25 and 35 pounds of cheese a year! Can you imagine? But when you think of all the cheeseburgers, pizza, grilled cheese, mac and cheese, cheesesteaks, cheesecakes, nachos, and queso dip we pour down our gullets, it is easy to believe. Much of the cheese we eat isn't about cheese, it is about texture. Americans crave fatty, salty goo. The French produce about 1,000 cheeses compared to the 400 produced in the United States, but theirs have more nutritional value than what we are cranking out. The amount of cheese we eat has tripled over the past 40 years, and cheddar does play a role in the rolls that are spilling over our belts. I love cheese more than the next guy, but I'm learning to treat my passion as a friend, not a lover. (Yes, I have taken cheese to bed, more than a few times.) Cheese can be a healthy choice, but it does depend on the type and the amount. Cheese is high in protein and calcium, both good things, but it also may be packed with sodium and saturated fats. Cheese has a bioavailability factor that is on our side, and it is a good source of calcium.

Cheese Rules:

Give up all processed cheeses—they are not cheese!

Try some nondairy cheeses made with almond, soy, and other dairy replacements. While not technically "cheese," they are healthy alternatives.

Organic and grass-fed cheeses are the best.

Choose non-GMO and hormone- and antibiotic-free cheeses.

Treat cheese like a condiment. Enjoy it with control. Preportion your cheese and don't go back for seconds.

Treat cheese like social drinking. Don't eat cheese alone!

(cha, cha, cha) chia seeds: Chia Pets were long the stuff of late-night TV commercials, but we now found that they can be an extremely healthy part of our diets! They may even have a link to healing diabetes.

This is another Mexican transplant that we should accept warmly at the border and welcome into our homes! Aztec warriors ate chia seeds to give them strength, energy, and endurance. Chia actually means "strength" in the Mayan language, and it was even used as currency. They are fiber rich and full of omega-3s, protein, vitamins, minerals, and antioxidants. In fact, some studies show that the natural phenolic compounds in chia may stop up to 70 percent of free radical activity. Chia seeds form a fiber gel in the stomach that can work as a prebiotic supporting growth of probiotics in your belly. These little antiaging seeds are good for your skin and help with digestive health, heart protection, and boost your energy and metabolism. To get the most from your chia, it is best to soak them (2 tablespoons to a cup of liquid for 2 hours or overnight) or grind them in a spice grinder or high-powered blender. Soaking them releases the enzyme inhibitors that protect the seed and makes them easier to digest, allowing the body to access the dense nutrients inside the seeds. Unlike flaxseeds, chia may be eaten whole and still allow you to enjoy the benefits, whereas the tough kernel on the flaxseeds prevents absorption.

chickpeas: We think of chickpeas as the bean that created hummus . . . but they have a much more interesting history! The wild chickpea has been tracked back to several countries in the Middle East, and some of those earlier varieties are still being used throughout the area, and in Asia, especially in India, where the darker peas are called channa.

chiffonade: Oh, those French . . . it is as if they have a descriptive word for everything! *Chiffonade* is one of the many knife cuts that every culinary student learns in the kitchen. It is basically a ribbon cut of leafy greens or herbs.

(red hot) chili peppers: Despite, or maybe for some because of their burning taste, chili peppers have long been considered a *healthy spice*. And some would say, an addictive drug! The capsaicin compound binds with pain receptors at the nerve endings that sense pain and cause pain and burning sensations without actually causing any bodily damage. This may help relieve pain in other areas of the body. This same reaction may aid in weight loss by tricking the brain by reducing appetite and increasing metabolism, which helps in fat burning. Chilies are especially popular in equatorial countries where the weather is hot. The chilies cause perspiration, which cools the body as it dries.

chinoise: This is a cooking tool that is used for straining liquids or thin purees. The French translation for *chinoise* is Chinese and was used to describe the cone-shaped colander that they believed looked like a Chinese hat. They come with various sizes of holes from large to mousseline, which is an extremely fine mesh.

cinnamon: As food for thought, cinnamon has been used medicinally for thousands of years, and modern science is now finally catching up. This spice is made from the inner bark of the cinnamon tree and has been regarded as a gift of the gods to the kings of ancient Egypt. Cinnamon outranks garlic and oregano in the amounts of antioxidants it contains. It also has important anti-inflammatory properties, helps the body to fight infections, and repairs tissue damage. It is touted as a cure-all for everything from diabetes, neurodegenerative diseases, cancer prevention and treatment, and bacterial and fungal infections to belly bloat, tooth decay, bad breath, and it even helps those with HIV. This wonder ingredient is even used to help preserve foods in many cultures. In short, don't just put it on your oatmeal.

cocoa: Chocoholics rejoice! However, not too fast. Cocoa has intrinsic health benefits from the flavonoids it contains. These antioxidant and anti-inflammatory functions have extremely positive health effects but with a catch! You must pick varieties that are low in added fats and sugars. The less sugar and dairy added to cocoa, the more you can really taste the quality and complexity of the bar. Compare it to drinking that sweet picnic wine or having a great Zinfandel. And, like wine, when consumed responsibly, it has some wonderful benefits. It can control free radicals, improve bad cholesterol levels, increase good HDL cholesterol, and lower blood glucose and LDL levels. Try adding cocoa powder to spice rubs, cocoa nibs to sweets, have a little dark chocolate on whole wheat toast with nut butter for breakfast, have a frozen banana dipped in dark chocolate and rolled in pumpkin seeds as a treat. Remember, if you are caffeine sensitive you might not want to take this to bed with you.

corn: I'm proud to be from corn country, and, yes, I have played more than my share of corn hole, but let's not get corny about this. Corn is good food. It is also 'Merican! And by that I mean Native American and Mexican. Can you imagine a world without grits, polenta, cornmeal, hominy, and corn on the cob? What is a movie without "air-popped" popcorn? As a healthy eater, I will encourage you to step outside of the box of corn flakes, try some new and interesting corn options, and give up on some of the corn "crack" that Americans have become addicted to. First of all, get off the GMO train and on to organics. Get all processed foods out of your pantry, including anything with corn syrup. Try different colored corn varieties. Remember that rainbow diet? Try "Indian," purple, red, blue, and pink kernels as well. They all have unique flavors. There is even a non-GMO orange corn being developed at Purdue University to be sent to countries where carotenoids are missing from the diet. Corn on the cob is a good source of fiber, and any time you eat a food you need to chew, it is satisfying and slows you down allowing you time to enjoy your meal.

crème fraîche: This is a rich, cultured heavy cream product used widely in France. Think of sour cream on steroids.

cruciferous veggies: Broccoli and its kin are some of the most eaten veggies in the United States, but few know just how nutritionally good they are for people! Broccoli in all its forms (sprouts, broccolini, broccoli rabe, and traditional florets) is a member of the cruciferous family, which includes all the cabbages, mustards, cauliflowers, collards, and many Asian greens like bok choy. All these are great bundles of antioxidants, anti-inflammatories, detox-support nutrients, and anticancer nutrients. The folic acid and vitamin C in crucifers help pregnant women with the DNA synthesis of the developing baby, helping to prevent birth defects. Calcium in these veggies helps to build bone mass. Its phytonutrients assist in detoxifying the body from alcohol and other chemicals. Finally, these veggies help keep the skin healthy and shining.

Types of Cruciferous Vegetables:
arugula
bok choy
broccoli
broccoli rabe
broccolini
brussels sprouts
cabbage
cauliflower
collards
horseradish

kale
kohlrabi
mustard greens
radish
red cabbage
rutabaga
turnip greens
turnips
watercress

cucumbers (Eat your water!): Cucumbers are one of the best ways to add more liquid to your diet. Between celery and cucumbers, it is a toss-up on which is the healthy eaters' best friend. They are the fourth largest cultivated "vegetable" in the world. Cucumbers are technically a fruit, and are in the same family as melons, squash, and pumpkins; but as far as ease of preparation cucumbers can't be beat. They add volume to your plate without adding many calories and have a satisfying crunch that makes your brain feel good. Although they may seem like a blank canvas as far as flavor goes, they still have a good deal of nutritional value with good amounts of vitamin K, B vitamins, copper, potassium, and vitamin C. They might even help prevent memory loss and some cancers. Cucumbers freshen your breath, cool the body's inflammation, and aid indigestion. Cucumber juice is a great base for any vegetable juice, and I love making cucumber water or cucumber lemonade on a hot summer day. Replace fatty chips with skinny cucumber disks the next time you want to get your dip on.

cumin (It's not just for Tex-Mex): Cumin is at the heart of many of the flavors of the Southwest and South of the Border, but its influence in the cuisines of the world reaches to almost every corner. Cumin only follows black pepper in popularity in the spice world. I have recently been discovering how much cumin is used in Chinese cooking and have fallen in love with Chinese cumin lamb. The iron in the spice helps maintain energy levels by improving blood flow and oxygen delivery. Lactating mothers often use cumin to assist in increasing breast milk supplies. Some studies show a possible protective effect from some cancer development. It has been used for digestive issues, diarrhea, and flatulence because of its levels of thymol, a good reason to add it to your beans the next time you make chili! Cumin is thought to increase the heat in the body, improving metabolism. It is also used in detoxification by improving kidney and liver operations and clearing waste and impurities through your urinary system. This last function also improves the skin by decreasing breakouts of acne, blemishes, rashes, and boils caused by toxins.

dried fruit: Eating one to two cups of fruit a day may seem like a lot, but if you just add some plums, figs, raisins, currants, dates, and figs you will find it easy to hit your mark. Remember dried fruits contain about five times the fiber in volume to fresh fruit, but drying also concentrates their sugars, creating a nice balance between fresh and dried.

eggplant: Black is beautiful! And so is purple, green, and white! *Aubergine* is the French term for this fabulous friend. Eggplant is great for those Meatless Monday meals, as it gives recipes "meatiness" and a filling quality. Eggplant is not just for Italian eggplant parm! In Thailand, the crisp small green eggplants give a crunch to spicy curries; in Japan, it is glazed with miso; in the Middle East, it is turned into tangy baba ghanoush. Eggplants are very rich in minerals, vitamins, and dietary fiber, which help keep your systems clean and firing on all cylinders. This will be evident through flawless, glowing skin. They may even help to prevent skin cancer. Speaking of cancer, eggplant has a small amount of nicotine and is suggested as a dietary supplement for people naturally quitting smoking cigarettes! On top of all that, it helps keep hair shiny and the scalp smooth (for those of us with receding "domes"). How to select one, you ask? Look for eggplants that have smooth, shiny skin, and bright color; that are heavy for their size and firm to the touch; and that have larger scars on the blossom end, because those will have the fewest seeds.

eggs: Almost the perfect package: It seems that every couple of years there are new thoughts on whether the egg is an angel or a devil. Well, as far as I'm concerned, we can settle that once and for all. The pastured chicken or duck egg is about the most perfect creation on Earth. Poultry that eat omega-3 rich clover, alfalfa, and insects can provide a good percentage of anti-inflammatory omega-3 fats to our diets. The problem with eggs is that they are very low in fiber, so eating eggs is fine as long as you enjoy them with high-fiber sidekicks.

Confusion on aisle 12!
In the supermarket egg section, this is what you might see:
cage-free
free-range
free-roaming
omega-3
omega-3 enriched
organic
pastured
pasture-raised

I suggest you buy your eggs from a local farmer whom you can look in the eye and ask questions about how his or her chickens are treated. I like my egg sunny-side up or poached soft, so I need the best and freshest eggs possible. But,

if you are unable to do this, I would go for the organic variety. Store your eggs in the refrigerator and try to use them within a week, two at the most.

EVOO: Cooks' slang for extra-virgin olive oil—the fat of the gods.

farro: What is old is new again. Farro, the wheat that has an ancient pedigree, is now the hottest thing since freekeh! Caesar and the gang loved farro for its toothsome earthiness and for being a cheap way to keep an army on the battlefields. But trendy things usually come down to taste, and I think farro is worth keeping around for more than a season. I love the undertones of sweet spices and the rich cashew-like mouthfeel. It is a 24/7 grain that finds itself comfortable at a black-tie event or at the breakfast table the next morning. Farro has the same benefits as most whole grains.

fermented foods: I'm in a pickle. Humans like to make the most of a good thing, and, when it comes to food, that means preserving it. Fermentation not only makes ingredients last longer, but it actually brings about chemical reactions that make foods beneficial to our bodies in new ways. Almost any food can be fermented in some way, but we are discussing veggies here. Think of kraut, kimchi, pickles, hot sauces, and vinegars. *Many fermented foods offer us higher nutritional value than the fresh.* For example, sauerkraut has more vitamin C than fresh cabbage. But the biggest nutritional value of these foods is in the probiotic content, which aids in digestive issues and nutrient absorption. Our ancestors' diets were full of probiotics, but ours are seriously lacking. Most of our food, even our pickles, is pasteurized. This makes us more susceptible to the grief unfamiliar bacteria cause us. Look for REAL fermented foods like kimchi, kavas, kombucha, and true kraut in the refrigerator of your local food co-op or health food store.

fish, shellfish (and other marine creatures): In general when we speak of fish we are suggesting that you try to find the best quality wild, sustainable, and humanely caught varieties. But there are alternatives to this rule and reasons why one may be unable to achieve the goal. First of all is price. Many of these products are extremely expensive. Second, unless you live in a large, affluent coastal city, it is likely that you wouldn't be able buy the best seafood even if you were a billionaire! Now, with the internet, you might be able to put your hands on wonderful ingredients if you are one who loves to plan ahead; but I'm sometimes thinking about Sunday dinner at 3:00 p.m. that afternoon. Also, there are some really good farm-raised sea and freshwater foods. Sustainably and ecologically farmed fish may help with the overfishing of our oceans and produce proteins that are healthy and nutritious for the mass market. Do your research and make sure that they are fed a proper, safe diet that you want to put in your body. Watch for artificial colors and waste products in feed. This concern is especially important when eating imported farm-raised products.

flaxseed: I have been adding a lot of flaxseed to my diet lately and I feel it has made a real difference in my body. I believe it has improved my general health and made me stronger against disease. It contains omega-3 fatty acids, vitamins E and B, calcium, iron, potassium, and antioxidants. I think eating or drinking flaxseed in a smoothie is the best way to get the most benefits, but you can take flaxseed oil in capsule form. Remember, when taking supplements you generally miss out on many of the other benefits of the ingredient such as fiber, and the body may not react to the supplement in the same way it does to the food source.

foraged foods: On the fertile Caribbean islands they have a saying that "ya can wake up with nothing and go to bed with a round belly." This means that if you know what you are doing, you can go into the woods and find all that you need to survive without spending any money. Well, it might be a little more difficult when you aren't on a tropical island, but, truth is, there is culinary gold in them thar hills! The Native Americans know this; how do you think they "got by" before Kroger grocery stores? From the first green sprouts of wild garlic mustard and onions, through mushroom and berry season, and finishing with persimmon and nut season, there is almost always something wild to eat. Most wild foods are more nutrient rich than domesticated foods. Yes, they are stronger in flavor, but where there is flavor, there are flavonoids.

Chef D's Top 10 List of Favorite Foraged Foods follows!

10. Cattails—pollen, cobs, roots
9. Spring greens!—nettles, dandelions
8. Nuts!—black walnuts, hickory nuts
7. Edible flowers—rose hips, day lilies, etc.
6. Wild garlic mustard greens
5. Wood sorrel
4. Wild garlic and onions
3. Stone fruit!—paw paws, persimmons, autumn olives
2. Berries!—blackberries, strawberries, raspberries, mulberries, service berries
1. Wild mushrooms!

A note on wild mushrooms from Chef D:
Never eat a mushroom that you are not 100 percent sure of. There are many look-alikes that can be deadly. There are many clubs and websites that may help, but it is best to have

the mushroom checked out by a local specialist.

freekeh (Get your freekeh on!): This ancient grain, centuries old, has been used throughout North Africa and the Middle East as a dietary staple. Freekeh is an heirloom wheat of the region that is harvested while still green and put through a roasting process that adds a nutty, smoky flavor. It is fairly quick-cooking, about 20 minutes, so it can be put on to simmer while you get the rest of your meal together. It is used as a side dish, cereal, pudding, pilaf, or even in soup, baked casseroles, and salads. Freekeh has three times the fiber of brown rice so it gives one the feeling of satiety, which is important when trying to cut down on calories. Freekeh can be found at ethnic stores and online and is becoming more available in health food stores and supermarkets. It is a wheat, so it is not gluten-free.

fresh (isn't always best!): Yes, fresh produce just picked by a local farmer or out of your own garden is always going to taste the best and have the most nutritional value; but there are many times that either our favorite foods are out of season or we are out of time putting a meal together. Oftentimes the produce at the local supermarket has been shipped in from California or Florida and may be days or even weeks old. These products are varieties raised for shipping, not for flavor, and others are picked before natural ripening and gassed to change their colors to be uniform and eye catching. Again, they're not the best thing for flavor. In those times, frozen is the way to go. Most frozen fruits and vegetables are harvested ripe with the highest amount of nutrition, flavor, and sweetness. They are processed and packaged very close to the time of harvest and are maintained at a nutrient-preserving temperature below

zero. Some frozen vegetables actually have more beneficial nutrients than fresh. For example, frozen peas have more beta-carotene than fresh ones.

garlic (Keeps vampires and doctors away!): There is only one negative to garlic and that is it gives you bad breath; other than that, it is a superfood! It is high in a sulfur compound called allicin, which is believed to bring most of the health benefits. To get the maximum benefit from garlic, it should be crushed and allowed to oxidize for several minutes or eaten raw. It is low in calories and very rich in vitamin C, vitamin B6, and manganese. It also contains trace amounts of various other nutrients. This "stinking rose" helps to prevent and reduce the severity of common illnesses like the flu and common cold. When eaten with gusto, garlic appears to help with blood pressure and can be as effective as regular medications. Some studies show garlic helps in lowering lead toxicity. The antioxidants in garlic protect cells from damage and aging and may reduce the risk of developing Alzheimer's and dementia. But, more importantly, garlic tastes awesome! It can be used in several forms such as raw, granulated, powdered, or paste, so it is easy to get the 2–3 cloves you need per day. You really can have garlic for every meal. And if you feed it to your loved ones, no one will know who has garlic breath.

gluten-free (GF) products: As a chef, I ask myself, "Is this a real thing?" I mean on a busy weekend night it seems that up to half of the clientele is battling with some sort of dietary restriction. The truth is, if you don't have a true allergy, such as celiac disease, you might be doing your body and your pocketbook a real disservice. Gluten free/fat free does not mean more nutritious. In many cases foods have less fiber and more fat, sugars, and sodium than traditional baked goods. You will most likely pay more. Most food industry and marketing folks add an increased price for items that must be special ordered or handled in a special manor. This is not to mention that people on these diets are willing to pay more for something marketed as gluten-free; and we know it. Many customers will buy a product or make a menu choice for GF foods even if there was never gluten in it in the first place (think gluten-free hummus)! Also, you may gain weight. If you are purchasing gluten-free foods—and the same holds true when buying fat-free foods—during the production of these products, ingredients are added to make them taste more like the original to satisfy your craving, but this strategy backfires in the long run. All that being said, looking at the amount of processed white flour in your meal plan is a good idea. Cutting battered and fried foods, cakes and cookies, buns and breads, pretzels and starchy snacks is all a part of making healthy choices. The key is, know why you are cutting these items from your diets and not replacing them with something just as bad (or worse). Do expand your pantry with new alternatives to the old standbys. For example replace traditional wheat pasta with sweet potato, black bean, rice, mung bean, and other types of noodles. This can be done throughout your culinary repertoire.

goji berries: Goji, or wolfberries, have been used throughout Asia as both medicine and food for centuries. The leaves, roots, bark, and berries are used in traditional medicine for liver diseases, longevity, headaches, coughs, fatigue, abdominal pain, and even infertility. The only problem with goji is that it may interfere with modern pharmaceuticals, so make sure you check with your doctor for possible side effects and allergies. But if you do get the go-ahead, you have a great new ingredient to incorporate into your cuisine. They are extremely high in antioxidants that aid in liver protection, controlling diabetes and cholesterol levels, reducing fatigue, and increasing brain activity.

greens: These plants are the tip of the iceberg of healthy eating. Leafy vegetables are the best things you can add to your diet to make it more healthful. Even if you start with the "gateway" green, iceberg lettuce, which has little nutritional value, at least you have done something. Americans eat about 17 pounds of the stuff on their burgers, tacos, and wedge salads per year. All greens are excellent sources of calcium, vitamins A, C, and K, potassium, and folate, but the darker the color, the greater the benefits. Try kale, collards, spinach, turnip greens, mustards, salad greens, wild dandelions, and cabbages to name a few. Remember, when you buy turnips, beets, and kohlrabi, you get two veggies in one. I even cook nice-looking radish tops. Usually the more aggressively flavored the green the more nutrients and compounds it contains. Wild greens like dandelions and mustards have a lot of taste that some find too strong. If you or your family don't like those flavors, try adding a little to other greens that will balance them out. Also, try a little sweetness, smokiness, and saltiness to make the dishes more palatable.

heirloom vegetables: Like an heirloom quilt, so too are many vegetable and fruit seeds, as well as plant starts. Much of the fresh produce offered to us in the supermarket is very different from what was offered a century ago. Heirloom varieties are grown from seeds that have been harvested without damage, selected for their vitality, look pretty, and ship well . . . not for flavor. One of the favorite foodie heirloom products is tomatoes, but look for heirloom beets, squash, beans, lettuce, herbs, and, of course, fruits as well.

hemp (It's not just for stoners anymore.): Hemp actually had a long and important relationship with humans, more as a textile and rope-making plant than as a drug or food. Hemp is available in many products now, from oils, dressings, and marinades to protein powders, power bars, and gluten-free flours. It has anticancer qualities and is a great source of fiber, antioxidants, and protein. Medical marijuana (hemp) has been shown to be helpful in many ways as well, but if it isn't legal in your state, plan a vacation.

herbs, fresh vs. dried: I don't think there is a choice between dried and fresh herbs. I always choose fresh, but I'm a food snob. The great thing about dried herbs is that you can keep them in your pantry for a year and they won't go bad. I can't tell you how many times I've seen expensive fresh herbs go into my compost at work or at home. When using fresh herbs you may generally add 4–5 times the amount by volume.

heritage livestock: Heritage animals are breeds of food animals that have fallen out of favor with farmers for many reasons, most often because turning a profit with them is more difficult. But visit your gourmet butcher or farmers' market, shop the internet, or go to the farm itself, and experience the difference. Heritage animals are usually grown on smaller farms and usually in a more organic and humane manner. They are usually pastured on grass and not fed as much industrially produced feed. Try heritage fowl, pork, beef, sheep, and small game like rabbit, quail, and pheasant.

honey (Oh, honey!): As one of humankind's oldest and sweetest pleasures, honey has become known as a superfood. Its flavonoids and antioxidants provide a shopping list of great things for our bodies, from helping to prevent cancers and heart disease, reducing gastrointestinal disorders, and improving muscle recovery time to regulating blood sugar and improving our skin. Honey has long been used in traditional medicine and now is accepted by the Western medical community for its antibacterial and antifungal qualities. Some raw honeys possess friendly bacteria that may explain many of its therapeutic properties such as its effectiveness on some burn victims. There are many types of honey throughout the world. They vary widely in flavor and color depending on the bees' environments and the types of vegetation they consume for nectar and pollen. Always choose pure and raw honey; refined honey loses many of its vitamins, minerals, and enzymes. Cooking honey at high temperatures also reduces its nutritional value. Honey is sugar, and like other sweeteners it is high in calories. Infants should never be given honey in the first year of life because it may contain spores that can cause infant botulism. The rest of us should use honey in moderation.

horseradish (Feel the burn!): Horseradish has been a favorite of mine since I was a wee boy. Mom used to take me to the downtown Indianapolis Market and one of the first things that hit you was the smell of the royal root! As a member of the flavorful *brassicaceae* family— which includes mustards, cabbages, and wasabi— horseradish fits in well. Although usually eaten in small quantities, it packs a powerful punch of nutritional value. Chemicals in the root can defend against microbes and bacterial infections such as listeria, E. coli, and staphylococcus. The fiber and protein stimulate satiety without adding any fat, so it is a perfect condiment for healthy eaters. The potassium in horseradish helps to regulate the passage of fluids and nutrients between cells, which can help both heart health and blood pressure. And as everyone knows, the stuff smells strong, but that is an attribute! If you have a cold, allergies, or stuffy nose, take a whiff and feel the stimulation as your congestion clears.

juicing: Juicing is a quick and refreshing way to add more vegetables to your diet, but it shouldn't be used in place of eating whole fruits and vegetables. It removes a majority of the fiber and in turn increases the amount of sugars in the gut without the fiber to slow it down. Try to add low-sugar/high-liquid fruit and veggies like cucumbers, greens, and celery to cut the sweetness and make your juices healthier. Always choose whole fruits and vegetables when possible.

mocktails (The new cocktail hour!): Whether you are a recovering alcoholic or just wanting to lose a few pounds or wake up feeling better in the morning, you don't have to miss out on "cocktail hour!" Yes, the feeling that alcohol gives us is freeing and exhilarating, but, at the same time, it is also calorie-filled and allows us to lose control of our goals. With proper planning one can either completely cut out alcohol, lower consumption, or just mix it up a bit.

Here are Chef D's Top 10 List of Adult Mocktails:

10. Agave lemon/lime sour
9. Tonic-ginger-soda with orange bitters
8. Verbena iced tea
7. Tomato juice cocktail
6. Raspberry vinegar fizz
5. Mint crush
4. Raw cranberry spritzer
3. Honey and lavender toddy
2. Kombucha
1. Kvass fermented beet juice

mousseline: A French culinary term meaning light and fluffy, or light as a pillow. Generally, mousselines are "lightened" with whipped cream and are time-consuming recipes with technical difficulties. There are now great ways to make them without the extra calories, expertise, and kitchen time.

(magic) mushrooms: Mushrooms are mostly water, but the small percentage that is not H_2O has been long revered as a wonder drug in Eastern medicine. The Chinese and Japanese believe that they are health altering additions to your diet. The most popular and widely available exotic 'shrooms are shiitake, enoki, maitake (hen of the woods), and oysters. These all have much more nutritional and chemical value than the standard Paris mushroom (button) or Italian portabella or cremini. Other mushrooms I suggest you getting to know are morels, chanterelles, puffballs, hedgehog, black trumpet, wine cap, sulfur shelf, porcini, and lobster. There are many more delicious and nutritious fungi out there, but there are others that can be dangerously poisonous, so always be confident in your choices.

nori: There are some things we fall in love with, socially acceptable or not, and some things we want to love but somehow can't find pleasurable. Seaweed is one of those things. Thankfully, nori is the Santana of seaweed: classic, a little different, tasty, and something you have to keep on the menu. Traditionally, we think of nori as the salty, earthy wrapper around sushi, but it has become so much more. It is low calorie, full of fiber, and a significant part of getting your plant-based amino acids and proteins in a vegetarian diet. If you aren't using table salt, nori has the iodine you need without the sodium, and if you aren't a banana fan, you can find your potassium here.

nutritional yeast: I use this mainly on my popcorn and "cauliflower popcorn" to add a buttery look and taste to my favorite snacks. But the nutritional value is much greater than you might think. It is a great veggie-based source of Vitamin B-12, which is essential for red blood cell production. It aids in regulating metabolism, which helps in mood and alertness. One daily tablespoon provides all the B-12 you need, so have it on your yogurt in the morning and you're done! It is high in folic acid, which is an important ingredient for infant health and for pregnant women.

nuts and nut butter: My favorite snack, especially when tossed with popcorn, nuts reduce heart attack risk, lower bad cholesterol, protect artery walls, aid in building strong teeth and bones, help in weight loss, lower blood sugar levels, help with brain functioning, and nourish the nervous system. A nut (or fifteen) a day keeps the mortician away.

orange (is the new black): Oranges and all citrus are a lot like life. They can be sweet and they can be sour. But when life gives you lemons, make a citrus vinaigrette. When I was growing up, every properly raised child was given a glass of orange juice to start the day, or in the 1960s, possibly Tang. We have learned a lot since then. We know that most processed and packaged fruit juices are basically pretty close to drinking sugar water. To maximize the nutritional benefits and get the complete value from citrus (and all juicy fruits), you need to eat them whole. We all know about the high levels of vitamin C in citrus, but citrus also contains flavonoids, fiber, folate, and potassium. Citrus may also reduce plaque formation in your arteries and improve blood circulation. Citrus is virtually a fat-free food that is relatively low in calories and high in moisture, making citrus a real energy booster. There are many types of citrus out there, so mix it up a bit. Try eating and cooking with kumquats, blood oranges, pomelos, ugli fruit, and darling clementines. Don't forget to use the *zest* of citrus as an ingredient as well. It contains the real "perfume" of the fruit. Grate it into sauces, vinaigrettes, batters, baked goods, and marinades.

organic: One hopes, the purest form of food available, grown without chemical fertilizers, pesticides, and synthetic enhancers. Generally believed to be healthier for humans than industrially grown meats, vegetables, grains, and fruits.

pepitas (pumpkin seeds): These imports from Mexico bring many well-known benefits with them. They are very hard workers and deliver magnesium, zinc, and plant-based omega-3s. The zinc may help the "fellas" with prostate health and the "babes" with hot flashes, headaches, joint pain, and other symptoms caused by menopause. These fiber-packed seeds exhibit anti-inflammatory properties and may even put you in a "turkey coma" from their non-animal tryptophan.

pomelo: One of the largest of the citrus fruits and one of the lesser known in the States, it is at least the size of a softball but usually more the size of a cantaloupe or honey dew melon. Pomelo has a bright green skin with a thick white pith surrounding flesh that varies from deep pink to light yellow. Pomelo is used in many Thai salad and Asian dishes where the juicy segments are divided into the individual capsules of Pomelo punch! This is really the king of citrus: aiding in weight loss, reducing muscle cramping, helping the immune system, lowering blood pressure, improving digestion, and, possibly, reducing cancer and signs of aging.

potatoes: Try picking smaller varieties of potatoes with more skin to starch ratio. Most of the nutritional value in potatoes is just below the skin. Avoid green potatoes that have grown too close to the surface of the ground.

provisions: The root of good health and a full belly—carrots, beets, sweet potatoes, celery root, parsnips, turnips, rutabaga, and much more. These veggies, called provisions in the Caribbean, are the staple of the diet in many cultures. The thicker the skin, the longer they can be kept in the pantry. They are full of vitamins, minerals, and antioxidants. They add natural sweetness to recipes as well as belly-filling fiber and starch that can turn a pot of weak broth into a dinner for the masses. Many are stored at room temperature and others can last weeks in the crisper drawer of your refrigerator.

purslane: This mostly wild herb completely destroys the old saying about making a silk purse out of a sow's ear! (Purslane, one of the plants known as pig's weed, has all the value of the best silk without the calories of pork rinds!) Speaking of fat, the amount of omega-3 fatty acids in purslane are some of the highest in the vegetable world. This slightly acidic succulent can be used raw in salads, tangy soups, and sexy garnishes for any meal of the day. This green goddess keeps your skin, teeth, bones, and brain young and excited.

quinoa: The Incan wonder food, these red, blond, or black seeds are not "true" grains but often replace grains in recipes when grains are not available, or for people who are allergic to gluten. It is one of the few plant foods that contains all nine essential amino acids. Making it a darling for vegetarians and folks wanting a more plant-based lifestyle. Quinoa is high in fiber, magnesium, B-vitamins, iron, potassium, calcium, phosphorus, vitamin E, and various beneficial antioxidants, thus making it one of the powerhouses in human nutrition. This seed is higher in fiber than most whole grains, so use it and use it often. The large amounts of the flavonoids quercetin and kaempferol make this plant's antioxidant health benefits numerous. This seed is one of the most nutritious and tasty ingredients on the planet. Eat it! A note about *kaniwa* ("ka-nyi-wa") the South American and African "mini grain" quinoa variety: Usually dark brown in color, use as you would use their bigger brother.

rice:

Chinese black rice (a.k.a. forbidden rice): I love the color of this rice and have been serving it for years as a breakfast cereal and in rice puddings, but I had no idea how healthy it was for us. The "black" color, which goes to dark purple when cooked, is actually the same natural color that blueberries and Acai berries have, and black rice offers the same chemicals responsible for those high amounts of antioxidants in berries that assist our bodies in flushing out the buildup of waste in our organs. Although still quite uncommon, "forbidden rice" as it was known when only Chinese emperors were allowed to have it, shouldn't be a stranger at your table.

brown rice: Second to black rice, this rice is the next best choice. My favorite brown rice is the short-grain variety, but I also like brown basmati, texmati, and long-grain brown. All white rice was once brown rice. Humans learned that by removing the side hull and bran and "polishing" brown rice into white rice it was more tender, cooked faster, gave quicker energy, and looked prettier on the plate. However this process removed proteins, thiamine, calcium, magnesium, fiber, and potassium while giving the eater an insulin boost. Brown rice moves more slowly through the body providing a longer source of energy. It is more toothsome and has a nice toasty flavor. Brown rice is great hot or cold in a salad.

wild rice: This seed of a freshwater dwelling grass isn't rice at all. It is native to the Great Lakes region and has been eaten by Native Americans for centuries. It is low in fat and high in protein, fiber, and the amino acid lysine. It is second only to oats as a grain-based protein source and contains thiamin, riboflavin, iron, and potassium.

ring molds: No, these aren't some type of beneficial fermented bacteria, they are tools of the restaurant trade. They can be as simple as a tuna fish can with the top and bottom cut out, 2-inch pieces of PVC pipe, or professionally made stainless steel versions. Ring molds are used to make those fancy round presentations that chefs like to do when showing off, but they also can help you when portioning your food at home and making dishes for special dinners.

rouille: This reddish yellow garlicky sauce comes from the south of France where it often is served with bouillabaisse or classic fish soup. The name comes from an old Provençal word meaning "rust," but there is nothing rusty about the flavors of this mayonnaise-like dip. Try it on raw or steamed vegetables, grilled fish, cold meats, and in salads.

seafood: Getting hooked on seafood. Canned fish is one of the quickest and healthiest meals you can prepare: perfect for that no-brainer lunch, snack, or light dinner. But be aware of some things when picking out your fish *du jour*. Realize that the smaller the fish, the fewer heavy metals and toxins they contain. Larger fish eat smaller fish and the fish at the top of the food chain usually contain the most toxins. Smaller fish usually have a higher percentage of fat. Fish fats contain the healthy omega-3 rich fatty acids, so, fish like herring, mackerel, sardines, and anchovies are good choices. Fish rich in fat usually are a little "fishier" in flavor. Larger fish like tuna are often commercially caught by huge trolling nets, which also catch other marine life such as dolphins, sea turtles, and seals; this waste of marine life is not a sustainable harvesting practice. Canned crab, smoked oysters, octopus, squid, and clams are other options for your SOTP (see below) pantry. White-fleshed fish, in particular, are lower in fat than any other source of animal protein.

sea vegetables: Momma always said, "Eat your SEA veggies!" We all need more sea vegetables in our diet. Sea vegetables are a natural source of iron and iodine, which aid in thyroid and immune system functioning as well as in controlling female estrogen levels. Japanese women who generally consume more sea veggies, especially kelp, have lower rates of several types of cancer. *Fucoidan* in seaweeds is a complex carbohydrate with powerful anti-inflammatory qualities that may help with blood flow, aches and pains, and digestive issues.

sesame (OPEN Ses-A-Me!): Sesame seeds come in several shades—white, black, and brown—and I love them all. Toasting any of these seeds brings out their flavor and gives added crunch to any dish. They are great whole, ground into paste, crushed into *za'atars* or Japanese rice topping, or baked into breads and pastry. Sesame oil, either cold pressed or the more aromatic toasted sesame oils, are also staples of my kitchens, both at home and in the restaurant. The zinc in sesame is essential in producing collagen, which gives elasticity to the skin for a more youthful appearance. For those eating a more plant-based diet, the seeds are a great source of protein, and magnesium, fiber, anti-inflammatories, and antioxidant enzymes.

shiso (a.k.a. *perilla* or even "beef steak") is known as a Japanese mint that is used to garnish American sushi platters. Shiso is much more important than the pretty green or purple leaf of garnish that you don't eat on your raw fish platter: it might even prevent food poisoning! It has an earthy, musty flavor that I love and might even have anti-inflammatory and cholesterol-lowering properties. It's higher in calories than many lettuce leaves, but that is because it contains healthy fats that many "greens" don't.

Szechuan pepper (prickly ash): This pepper is not a pepper, it is actually the dried flower bud of an Asian prickly ash tree. It is used in Szechuan cuisine for its numbing effect, which is considered a "seventh" flavor. Try it in small amounts and see how you like it. I love it!

sorghum: The molasses of the midwest, Sorghum is both a grain and a thick syrup made from the reduction of the sap made from squeezing the stalks of the grassy plant. The seed can be used as a grain and cooked whole like a cereal or ground like a grain. The thick, rich syrup can be used for sweetening in the same manner as maple, honey, cane, and other syrups.

SOTP (a.k.a. "sautéing off the pounds"): These are recipes that all readers can use to introduce themselves to creative and healthy ways of cooking and eating.

soy and soy products (miso paste/soup): Soy, oh boy. One of my favorite snacks, other than pistachios, is edamame. I was first turned on to this by my Japanese chef friends twenty or so years ago. Those beans were unfamiliar, tasty, nutritious, and delish! Edamame are fresh, tender, green Japanese soy beans. They are traditionally served in their pods with sea salt as a bar snack or appetizer. Now you can buy edamame in most Asian markets and even in a lot of big box stores either in their pods or shelled, and also frozen for use in many recipes. As with most beans, they are a powerhouse of vegetarian protein, packed with fiber, vitamins, and minerals.

squash (summer and winter): Summer squash are basically yellow squash or zucchini. There are other kinds in various shapes and colors, but they can all be used pretty much interchangeably. They are low in calories, and, because they are fairly bland, they are good vehicles for many stronger flavors like garlic, tomatoes, and basil. They are thin-skinned and high in moisture, making them highly perishable and in need of refrigeration. Winter squash come in a huge variety of sizes, shapes, colors, and textures. They have much less moisture than their summer cousins and a much thicker and more protective tough, exterior skin. They are used throughout the world and have fed the human brain in every non-arctic culture for millennia. Giant wedges of yellow and orange squash are sold throughout Africa, South America, Asia, and the Caribbean for use in soups and stews. In America, we use them in both savory and sweet recipes. They are high in fiber, vitamins, and minerals. The many varieties have the ability to improve bone and skin health, strengthen the immune system, build strong bones, hearts, and eyes, eliminate parasites, reduce blood pressure, and ease arthritis. They might even help you get a better night's sleep. So mix it up and do some research. Every type of squash is like a healthy prescription. The only downside is that some are so effective in lowering blood pressure that folks with hypotension should avoid them.

sriracha: If you can't stand the heat . . . leave off the sriracha (a.k.a. rooster sauce). Named after the Thai village of Sri Racha, this American sauce was created in the '80s by a Vietnamese immigrant who couldn't find a hot sauce in the States that met his liking. It is a favorite in most restaurant kitchens as well, and there is usually a bottle out on the table during staff meal period no matter if it is breakfast, lunch, or dinner. It is a blend of red chilies, garlic, vinegar, salt, and sugar and can really "bring up" the flavor of a bland dish with just one squirt.

sweating: This culinary term describes a method of cooking using gentle, moist heat. Mostly used for recipes beginning with onions and/or garlic, sweating is cooking without coloring or caramelizing the ingredients.

tagine: When we speak of this dish we are generally referring to the Moroccan version. This North African dish is a wonderful balance of sweet, spicy, and fragrant flavors. The name comes from the cooking vessel that looks something like a terracotta UFO. In a land of little water, long-cooked dishes must retain their moisture through human ingenuity. The cone-shaped top gathers the natural moisture of the cooking process and returns it to the lower rimmed cooking plate.

tahini paste: This is basically sesame seed "butter" and is used throughout the Middle East, India, and Asia in both savory and sweet recipes. Tahini is what puts the "hum" in hummus! Sesame seeds are rich in iron, copper, manganese, and calcium. Note: Also try black and white sesame seeds for the same health benefits. When using whole sesame seeds, try toasting them in a dry pan until they smell toasty. This method brings out their rich flavors and adds a more crunchy texture to your recipe. They are a great topping for rice, salads, and many veggie dishes.

Tajin clasico salsa con polvo, con limon: This shakable sour, sweet, and spicy spice blend can add a blast of flavor hitting every taste bud in your mouth. Try it on just about anything south of the border from cocktails to fresh fruit.

tamari vs. classic Chinese soy sauce: Tamari is an alternative Asian umami flavoring sauce that is extremely important in the healthy vegetarian and vegan kitchen. Tamari also has a home in the SOTP pantry. It generally is thicker in viscosity, less salty in flavor, and can be gluten-free. Make sure you check the labels, though. Some versions do contain a small fraction of wheat. Use in stir-fry, sauces, vinaigrettes, dips, marinades, and brines.

teff: This is the grain that the famous Ethiopian sour dough crepes are made out of. These giant but very thin "pancakes" are served with a huge variety of stews and braises and take the place of silverware at the table. If you ever get the chance, you must go to an Ethiopian restaurant!

tempeh: My love affair with tempeh has been warming up as of late. I like to purchase varieties that have added flax and other ingredients. My favorite way to cook it is to dice it up, sauté it until GBD (golden brown and delicious), and toss with chopped garlic, capers, and flat-leaf parsley.

tomatoes, the 24/7 veggie: The lycopene in tomatoes is nature's natural sunblock and the vitamin A helps with night vision, so you should be eating these babies all day long. They are packed with vitamin C, low-cal, fat-free, high in fiber and water (so they make you feel full), and they help regulate your blood sugar. To get more of the red stuff in your meal plan, enjoy them in huevos rancheros for breakfast, fresh on sandwiches and salads at lunch, by the handful as a morning or afternoon snack, or in sauces, stews, and soups at dinner. Oh, and an occasional Bloody Mary at brunch!

tomatoes, canned: Nothing beats the can-can—the Moulin Rouge of food—like tomatoes. Canned tomatoes offer something that fresh can't. Tomatoes are preserved using heat, which releases lycopene—this carotenoid may help prevent some cancers. Canned tomatoes are often already peeled, chopped, and ready to use in cooking. When packed in glass jars or aseptic boxes, in addition to BPA-free cans, they are recipe ready. This is one example where canned wins over fresh.

tropical fruit: Most fruits grown on or near the equator are extremely exotic and sweet-smelling. This makes them very attractive to our taste buds, but the hot regional sun also packs them full of sweet sugars making them a treat to eat in limited quantities.

TVP (textured vegetable protein): This should be every healthy cook's buddy. It is easy to use, lasts a long time in the cupboard, and adds protein without fat or cholesterol. It comes in several forms from larger "meaty" stew-like chunks, to more of a ground meat size, and even a "flour-like" powder. It is great in tomato sauces, curries, stews, and even sauces and smoothies. It is rich in dietary fiber, folate, and potassium, and low in sodium and fat, making it a great addition to your pantry.

Umeboshi paste (pickled plum paste with shiso): This is a great condiment that has a sweet, sour, and salty umami flavor. It is great in dressings and sauces or even on top of deviled eggs.

vinegars: There are so many types of vinegar available from different fruits to others infused with herbs, chilies, spices, and fruits. Vinegar adds an acidic kick to any dish and helps you cut salts and sugars from recipes. The Italians even serve strawberries with balsamic vinegar for dessert.

Wakami seaweed: Wakami is served in many Japanese miso soups and other dishes flavored with sesame and scallions. Like nori paper, it is fairly mild in flavor so I consider it a gateway seaweed.

wood ear mushroom: This strange looking black and crinkled fungus is most commonly found in Asian restaurants and markets. Once soaked and trimmed of the tough "foot," they add great texture to many soups, stir-fries, salads, and stews. Their chewy and slightly crunchy texture can replace meat in vegetarian recipes.

yogurt: This fermented dairy product is a healthy eater's friend. I especially like the richness of Greek-style, labneh, and kefir yogurts. As always, grass-fed pastured dairy products are best when available. Yogurt is full of good-for-the-gut live and active bacteria and probiotics that aid digestion and strengthen your immune system.

Za'atar (the "king of condiments"): In the Middle East, za'atar is a highly flavored dried blend of sour red sumac powder, thyme, oregano, marjoram, toasted sesame, and salt. Although available "over the counter," I feel homemade versions are fresher and give more of a "pop" to your recipes. You can also balance the equation to suit your own taste. Once you get za'atar in your kitchen you will find 101 ways to use it. I love it on flatbread, hummus, and yogurt dips, grilled vegetables, meat, fish, potatoes, eggs, just about everything but ice cream!

Za'atar

Ingredients:

¼ cup sumac, available at international markets

2 tablespoons dried thyme

1 tablespoon sesame seeds, roasted

2 tablespoons marjoram

2 tablespoons dried oregano

1 teaspoon coarse sea salt or Himalayan pink salt

½ teaspoon cracked black pepper

Pinch of red pepper flakes

Directions:

Pulse the sesame seeds in a blender, food processor, or with a mortar and pestle. Add the remaining ingredients and pulse. Do not overwork; it should be coarse.

Place in an airtight container. Stored in a cool dark space, za'atar can last several months. Actually, just leave the stuff on the counter so you remember to use it all the time!

INDEX

Page numbers in italics refer to photos.

237

Born in Southern Indiana of Polish, Scottish, and German blood, **DANIEL ORR (a.k.a. CHEF D)** feels that there must be a French showgirl somewhere in his heritage. His love for all things French led him to youthful follies throughout France and Belgium, working in seven Michelin-starred restaurants and engaging in his passions for Impressionist art, Parisian jazz, and pastis.

In the life-altering days after 9/11, he left his beloved Big Apple and his *NYT*'s 3-star position at La Grenouille and "Esquire Magazine's Best New Restaurant in America" post at Terrence Conran's Gaustavino's. He headed to the Caribbean paradise of Anguilla to work with Cuisinart's Brand-Maker Lee Rizzuto. He created his *Paradise Kitchen* methods of cooking with island fish, wild herbs, tropical fruit, and island "provisions."

Returning then to Indiana, he fell in love with the bounty of the Midwestern pantry. The nostalgia of his boyhood foraging and family gardening are now a part of his current cooking style, which blends farmstead ingredients with exciting global flavors at his restaurant, FARMbloomington, in Bloomington, Indiana.

Reaching his late 40s and early 50s, Chef D found that his passion for food, wine and bourbon were having an effect on his figure and his medical charts. Always looking for ways to cook healthy foods for his guests *and* himself, he began taking notes on his experiences. Meeting Dr. K in 2015, he asked her to help him with the battle of the bulge, and they developed the war plans that led to the *Wellness Lifestyle* plan.

DR. KELLY JO BAUTE (a.k.a. DR. K) is owner of A Splendid Earth Wellness and considers herself a total movement geek. She has over 20 years of experience in the health/fitness industry, from group and personal fitness instruction to health/fitness programming and administration. Unable to rest her curiosities about human movement, Dr. K pursued a unique combination of academic and research training and earned her doctorate in kinesiology (motor control and learning) and biological anthropology (functional morphology). Her research experiences include observational data collection of farm laborers' working postures in rural Dominican Republic; investigating recreational behaviors of eco-tourists in South Africa; and designing and conducting experimental lab investigations and simulations of motor behavior using electromyography, motion capture, and force plate data while using a stability ball as an office chair. Goals of her work include identifying postural and environmental indicators for risk of musculoskeletal injury; characterizing contemporary musculoskeletal adaptations and the associated evolutionary implications; and developing and disseminating preventative, corrective exercise interventions for functional issues.